Draw Me a Picture

DRAW ME A PICTURE

The meaning of children's drawings and play
from the perspective of the analytical psychology

Theresa Foks-Appelman
creative arts therapist

This book contains illustrations that were downloades from the internet. Written permission was given to use most of the illustrations; however, it was not always possible to trace the owner of a website or an illustration. For clarity's sake, all the internet illustrations are accompanied by the names of the related websites, and this information is also given in the literature list. If the author has used illustrations that are subject to copyright, the owner of the illustration(s) is requested to contact the author.

The case illustrations contained in this book have been taken from the author's practice. Although authentic, the names and the presenting symptoms have been altered to provide complete anonymity.

Original Dutch title: "Kinderen geven tekens. De betekenis van kindertekeningen vanuit het perspectief van de analytische psychologie." door. Uitgeverij Eburon te Delft, the Netherlands. First paperback printing, 2004; second printing, 2004, third printing, 2005.

English translation by Susan Parren-Gardner 2006/2007

Foxap scriptus, Nuenen the Netherlands
www. foxap.scriptmania.com
www.kindertekeningen.info
t.foks@onsnet.nu

ISBN 1-4196-6201-5
EAN 13: 978-1-4196-6201-0

Cover design: Geert Hermkens, *Studio Hermkens*, Amsterdam
(drawing cover Martin Gocobachi, 9 years old –(2001)

© 2007. Th.L.M. Foks-Appelman All rights reserved. No part of this publication may be reproduced, stored in a retrieval system, or transmitted, in any form or by any means, electronic, mechanical, photocopying, recording, or otherwise, without the prior permission in writing from the proprietor.

To my children and grandchildren

Jelle
Renate
Marijne
Jorik

CONTENT

Acknowledgements   xi

Preface to the English edition   xiii

CHAPTER 1   THE HISTORY OF DRAWING   1
- 1.1 The art of drawing   1
- 1.2 The first signs of life   2
- 1.3 The language of symbols   4
- 1.4 The meaning of a symbol   6
- 1.5 Symbols in art and religion   8

CHAPTER 2   THE PSYCHE AND THE ART OF DRAWING   11
- 2.1 The unconscious as a psychological phenomenon   11
- 2.2 The meaning of the mother archetype   12
- 2.3 The child and mythology   14
- 2.4 Body and psyche   17
- 2.5 Healing art   20

CHAPTER 3   DRAWING AND PSYCHOLOGY   25
- 3.1 Developmental psychology and the first years of childhood   25
- 3.2 The separation-individuation theory   26
- 3.3 Psychological research on children's drawings   29
- 3.4 Playing and therapy   32
- 3.5 Drawing and therapy   33
- 3.6 Jungian analytical therapy   34
- 3.7 Sandplay therapy   34

CHAPTER 4   CHILDREN'S FIRST DRAWINGS   37
- 4.1 Universal drawings   37
- 4.2 The drawing without borders   38
- 4.3 The egg-shaped drawing   40
- 4.4 The snake-like drawing   43
- 4.5 The spiral drawing   45

	4.6	Children who do not draw	46
	4.7	Ego-consciousness and the Self	47
	4.8.	The circle	50
	4.9	Sunrays	53
	4.10	Dots	56
	4.11	Crosses	59
	4.12	Balloons	61
	4.13	Coloured areas	64
	4.14	Smearing and messing about	65
	4.15	Colouring in pages of a colouring book	67

CHAPTER 5   **CHILDREN DRAW THEMSELVES**   69

	5.1	The significance of the tadpole	69
	5.2	Tadpole	71
	5.3	Tadpole with a belly	73
	5.4	Head and rump	74
	5.5	The pre-school child and magical thinking	76
	5.6	Details in drawings of human figures	78
	5.7	Learning to look at a drawing of a human being	87
		Case illustration 1	88
		Case illustration 2	91
		Case illustration 3	93

CHAPTER 6   **DRAWINGS OF HOUSES AND TREES**   95

	6.1	The symbolism of the house	95
		1. The round house	97
		2. The square house	97
		3. Details of a house	98
		4. The surroundings of a house	99
	6.2	Learning to look at a drawing of a house	103
		Case illustration 1	103
		Case illustration 2	105
	6.3	The symbolism of the tree	106
		1. The trunk	108
		2. Roots	108
		3. Animals	108
		4. Fruit	109
	6.4	Learning to look at a drawing of a tree	109

		Case illustration 1	110
		Case illustration 2	111
		Case illustration 3	112
CHAPTER	**7**	**CHILDREN CAN DRAW EVERYTHING**	**113**
	7.1	The latency phase (7 to 10 years old)	113
	7.2	X-ray drawings	114
	7.3	Drawings with a story	115
	7.4	Cartoons and trick drawings	117
	7.5	Spontaneous drawings	117
	7.6	The rainbow	118
	7.7	Traumatic events	118
		A child draws the war	120
	7.8	The period of group awareness	121
	7.9	Drawings by boys and drawings by girls	122
	7.10	Drawings of boats	124
	7.11	Aggression in children's drawings	126
	7.12	Depression in children's drawings	128
CHAPTER	**8**	**ADOLESCENTS DRAW THEIR OWN LINES**	**129**
	8.1	Puberty (10-15 years)	129
	8.2	Rituals of transition	131
	8.3	Contemporary rituals	132
	8.4	Music and dance in puberty	133
	8.5	Problems in puberty	134
	8.6	Drawing in puberty	136
		1. A new perspective	136
		2. Fantastic and surrealistic	137
		3. Cartoons	137
		4. Black and white drawings	137
		5. Drawing with feeling	138
	8.7	Children's drawings on the W.W.W.	138
	8.8	Giving up drawing	139
		Case illustration	140
CHAPTER	**9**	**COLOURS, FORMS AND LAYOUT**	**141**
	9.1	The symbolic significance of colours	141

	9.2	Psychological investigations into colour	142
	9.3	Colours and alchemy	149
		Case illustration	150
	9.4	The symbolic meaning of the basic forms	151
		1. The square	151
		2. The triangle	153
		Case illustration	154
	9.5	The symbolic significance of the layout	154
	9.6	Learning to look at the layouts of a drawing	157

CHAPTER 10 ANIMALS AND FANTASY FIGURES 161

	10.1	The animalistic phase	161
	10.2	The symbolic significance of animals	162
	10.3	Stuffed animals as transitional objects	166
	10.4	Why (stuffed) animals can help	167
	10.5	The significance of fantasy figures	169
		1. Elves	171
		2. Fairies	172
		3. Witches	173
		4. Magicians	174
		5. Dwarves	175
		6. Clowns	176

CHAPTER 11 INTERPRETING DRAWINGS 179

	11.1	Learning to look at children's drawings	179
	11.2	Drawings and signals	179
	11.3	Learning to look systematically	181
		1. Jung's typology	182
		2. The theory of phases and iconology	183
		3. The appeal analysis	184
		4. Investigating the symbolic significance	185
	11.4	Let me draw you a picture	186

REFERENCES 187

INDEX 193

Acknowledgements

I would like to thank the following people:

All those parents and children who gave me drawings to use in this book.

My family Ellen Roos, Karin de Bruin and friends Leonie van der Linden and Ineke Verrijk who supported me with their encouraging words and constructive criticism.

My daughter Renate who entrusted me with her children (my grandchildren) Marijne and Jorik one day a week, a day that I was free to enjoy while watching them playing and drawing.

My mother, who, even at the age of 100, was still interested in my work. She is the example of the 'Archetypal Mother' who nurtured and protected her large family. She died in 2005 at the age of 102.

My husband Nico Foks for his technical support at the computer and in processing the illustrative material.

Mary Jane Markell, founding member of ISST and a teacher of Sandplay therapy. Her years of experience as a child psychotherapist, her expertise and her intense love of children inspired me to write this book.

And last but not least, Susan Parren-Gardner for her enthusiastic and conscientious translation of my book into English.

Theresa L.M. Foks-Appelman
Nuenen, December 2006

Preface to the English edition

This book about the meaning of children's drawings first appeared in the Netherlands in 2004. Within two years, the third edition had been published and various universities for professional education (HBO in the Netherlands) had put the book on their reading lists. In addition to specialized books about the therapeutic use of drawing, there was a need for more clarity about the origins of the normal development of a child's drawings. Why do children make the same drawings about the same subjects? And why do adolescents stop drawing? A plan was launched to make this book accessible to a wider audience by publishing an English translation.

In this English edition, some paragraphs have been omitted from the text because they deal with typically Dutch subjects or refer to Dutch literature that has not been translated and that is not relevant for an international public. Moreover, some additions have been made to chapter 5 that did not appear in the third Dutch addition. And an index has been included in the English edition.

When my own children were still small, I first saw how children's drawings were made. I can still remember how surprised I was when I saw the first tadpole that my nearly two-year-old daughter had drawn on a piece of scrap paper. I was amazed and moved, and I have saved that drawing. My children later gave me more drawings, all of them wonderful. I somehow knew that children drew in the same fashion, but I did not know why. After studying art and psychology and receiving my diploma as a creative therapist from Utrecht University for Professional Education, I followed courses in Sandplay Therapy (according to D. Kalff's methodology) and I began to work in my own practice for child therapy with children and young people. I developed a course about the meaning of children's drawings, gave workshops to students from various institutes of pedagogics and held readings about children's drawings at parents' evenings at schools. The questions and comments from students, parents and teachers made me delve even deeper into the material available. Parents often asked me if I could see something in a drawing made by their child. It seemed as if they
suspected that a drawing revealed something about the child. I often

examined a drawing together with a parent, and I noticed that I saw much more in the drawing, not because I had a crystal ball but because I had insight. In principle, this insight can be developed by everyone.

To understand the deeper meaning of children's drawings, I began to search for the origins of art. The books by Erich Neumann, a Jungian analyst, were especially useful in providing me with the insight that a child repeats not only the biological history of his or her predecessors but also the history of the psyche. This could explain the universal development of the psyche of children, which is expressed in the ways in which children play and draw.

The insights provided by Carl Gustav Jung and later similar thinkers such as Erich Neumann, Ingrid Riedel, Marie-Louise von Franz and Rose Fleck-Bangert were important sources for my study of the deeper meaning of children's drawings. In my description of the meaning of children's drawings, a connection is made between the origin and developments of the expressive art of our predecessors and the origin of children's drawings. The significance of mythological stories and fairy tales for the psychological development of the child is connected to modern theories of developmental psychology.

This book is not a therapy manual. Using drawings in a therapeutic process requires special knowledge and skills and cannot be done without the necessary training and experience. However, psychologists, psychotherapists, creative therapists, other care providers and, of course, parents interested in the psychological development of their children can find support in the subjects dealt with in this book. All of them can profit from first learning about the psychology of the normal, healthy child who draws and plays before they begin to notice deviations in children's drawings as signals or signs. As a therapist who plays with children to help them become a child again, I am repeatedly impressed by a child's energy and creativity. By nature, children have access to a creative source; children with problems or in difficult circumstances show me again and again that there is a healthy core. For me, playing and drawing are a return to the paradise of childhood. I would like to invite the reader to come with me.

Theresa Foks-Appelman

CHAPTER 1

THE HISTORY OF DRAWING

1.1 The art of drawing

If asked to make a drawing, most children begin to draw spontaneously. They usually enjoy drawing, both at home and at school and together with other children. They think of a subject themselves or they copy something. They often make a drawing for a special occasion. Who of us does not remember the drawing for Mother's Day or for grandmother in hospital? When children are involved in especially traumatic experiences, adults often do not know what they can do to help the child. It can be a relief to a child if you say, 'Would you like to draw something about what happened'? Drawings by children living in a disaster area or a war zone are always impressive and moving to see because, in these sorts of drawings, children tell us how terrible the experience was and how afraid they were. Then we do not have to ask, 'How did you feel'? The child shows us the scene in question and we look at it together with them; we are witnesses to that awful moment and to what the child experienced.

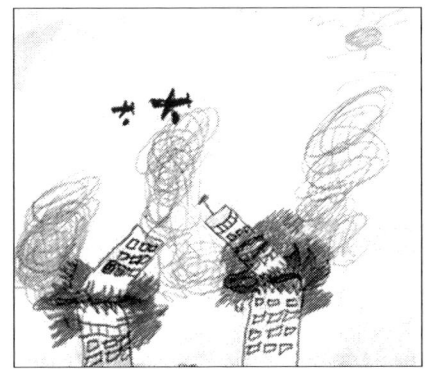
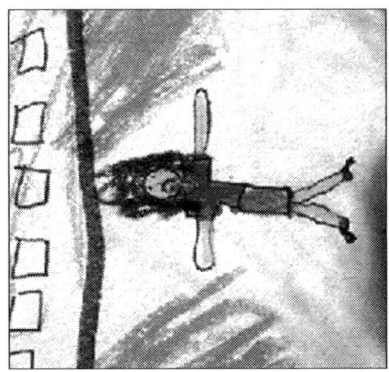

Drawing by boy (9 years old)
depicting New York
11 September 2001

This ability to spontaneously express an inner feeling is common to all children up to a certain age. Adults are able to do the same (again) if they find themselves in a difficult situation, for example, when confronted with a serious illness or loss. Artists are able to do so by their nature, drawing on a source of inner inspiration. Some artists can make drawings that often cause people to say, 'My child can do that too', as if it were 'nothing'. But is it not very special that, by nature, children are able to make drawings that only a few artists are also able to create? Every adult was once an artist, but this talent disappears in most of us. Or perhaps we still have the talent but we are no longer able to call it forth? I will return to this issue of art and ability later in this book.

1.2 The first signs of life
Let us go back in time and look at why humans began to draw. We can imagine that our ancestors, when coming to a crossroads on their way to their hunting grounds, drew a line with an object or perhaps even placed a cross on a rock or a tree. They did this both for themselves so that they could find their way back home and for others to show them which way to go. The sign meant 'I was here'. It was a trail that people left behind them as they went, proof that they had reached a certain point.

Leaving behind signs is of great importance in the development of the human psyche. There was a time in the history of human development, although we do not know exactly when, when our ancestors were very closely connected to nature and their instincts as they wandered across this planet to look for food here, something to drink there. Sleeping, sexual intercourse and reproduction were natural events that primitive man did not stop to reflect on. It was a sort of earthly paradise in which people lived without thoughts, imagination or responsibilities. People were unconscious of themselves. We can assume that no single man or woman one day suddenly said, 'I think, therefore I am', but rather that, differing per individual, early man gradually 'saw a light' and slowly became aware of 'a feeling'. Individuals slowly became conscious of the fact that they 'were on a road' and 'were travelling to a destination'. Expressing this in the form of a sign gave a certain support to this consciousness.

Recognizing a written sign is an intellectual activity. There are indications that certain sorts of animals, such as apes, dolphins and horses, are also able to recognize drawn symbols, something that should not surprise us because these animals are known to be intelligent and closely associated to human beings. However, there is no proof that animals can draw symbols themselves, let alone think of them. The signs enabled long-distance communication between human beings. The possibility of making contact with another human who was not present at that moment but who might recognize the sign at a later moment meant that the human psyche was capable of remembering another person.

Memory is a complex intellectual system. As children develop psychologically, they are able to identify and recognize a person or an object. For a long time, children do not know that a person (or a thing) continues to exist even when they do not see it. A child is surprised again and again when someone whom he or she loves comes into view. For example, if the mother has left the room, the child will search in his or her immediate surroundings but, if the mother cannot be found, the child will stop searching or will begin to cry. The child's brains are not yet capable of thinking that someone or something could be somewhere else. That is also why a child of one and a half or two cannot understand that a mother's voice on the telephone means that she is elsewhere. The child responds to the mother's voice but is not comforted if she says 'I'll come to get you soon' or 'I love you'. The child needs the mother's physical presence to believe that the mother really exists. In the course of a child's third year, the brains become capable of remembering an image (or a person) as an object, the so-called 'constant object' as described by the British researcher *Bowlby*. Similar results were also described in *Piaget's* theory which refers to this sort of memory as the 'assimilation phase'.

The appearance of a sign, the predecessor to a real drawing, shows that human beings began to develop intellectually and to move a step closer to becoming conscious. In the same way, children will begin to draw only as they begin to develop intellectually and are able to give a (symbolic) word to the meaning of people, things and thoughts. A drawing is a symbol of communication that demands a certain form of self-consciousness. Between the ages of one and a half and three, children become increasingly aware of both themselves and those around them. They make their first scribbles especially for themselves, but drawings are gradually used to communicate. Children who have a contact disorder are capable of copying an object onto paper, but they find it difficult, if not impossible, to make a spontaneous, imaginative or symbolic drawing.

The earliest form of human communication in drawings that we know of consists of drawings on clay tablets and stones or sculptures made from clay, wood or stone. They transmit a message, a wish or a thought that is expressed in symbols. Examples of prehistoric drawings are cuneiform script, hieroglyphics and the famous cave drawings. In the past few decades, researchers have investigated the meanings of these drawings. Because children are still in close contact with the symbolic language of drawings, it is useful to examine the history of this language.

1.3　The language of symbols

The word 'symbol' is derived from the original Greek meaning of the word *sym-bolon* = 'throwing together'. There is a story that, at dinners in ancient times, two people broke a gnawed bone (e.g. a chicken leg) in the middle; each saved his or her half so that, if they (or their descendants) met again, they would 'throw' the pieces of bone 'together' as a symbol of recognition and brotherhood. They called their piece of bone a *symbolon* (*H.R. Graetz*). This story involves a visible, tangible object and an invisible expression of feeling.

The first psychologists to examine the meaning of symbols were Freud and Jung in the early 20th century. Freud considered symbols in dreams as expressions or fulfilments of unconscious wishes, most of which he said were sexual. It was the analytical psychologist Carl Gustav Jung who searched for a more extensive and deeper meaning of symbols. He discovered universal forms that appeared in drawings from earlier times and cultures and that point to universal meanings. Impressions, ideas and events in nature that we cannot understand completely are represented in symbols (C.G. Jung, *Man and his symbols*). Jung called some of these forms, contents and symbols 'archetypes'.

One of the oldest examples of a symbolic meaning attached to a natural object is the stone. The symbolism of the stone has always fascinated mankind because the stone is the rudimentary material of the earth, a material that has always existed and that always will. That is why, in symbolic language, a stone is referred to as the alchemist's stone or the philosophical stone because a stone contains the past, the present and the future. People once believed that gods and spirits resided in stones, which is why, in primitive cultures, people placed stones on graves. This gave stones a special symbolic significance. Gravestones are still a symbol of remembrance. Even today, modern sculptors choose a stone by trying to see what is hidden in the stone.

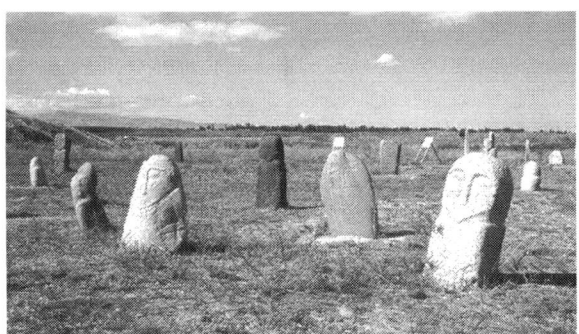

(Gravestones. Kochto. Oezbekistan) photo S. Gheraert

It is interesting to note that, as in the past, both girls and boys continue to collect stones. Stones have an attraction; people want to save them, touch them or keep them in a special place. It is remarkable that the first book in the globally popular Harry Potter series is entitled *The Sorcerer's Stone*. The author J. Rowling used an old symbol in her modern language, which was suited to the present and understood by so many children.

In the contemporary world in which the written word has become so very important in the form of books, newspapers and computers, we nevertheless see the need to use symbols – pictures that everyone can recognize – to communicate our messages. Nothing makes a message clear as quickly as an uncomplicated, strong symbol. Think of the many icons used in computer and word processing programmes to clarify the use of the various functions. Drawn images are also increasingly often used in international human traffic at, for example, airports, in restaurants, at tourist attractions, etc. However, these are signs that have been thought of by the intellect and that usually have no deeper significance.

In children's games, dreams and stories, modern images can have a symbolic meaning. For example, if a child draws or dreams of a plane, the plane can be the modern representative of the symbol 'bird'. A plane can fly like a bird and even looks like a bird. But a plane also has other dimensions: explosive force, energy and noise. A plane also signifies adventure, discovery, visits to other countries, the need to have a proof of identity, luxury, holidays and global contacts, so that a plane has become a new, modern symbol.

A symbol is an archetypal form of expression with a dynamic aspect; a symbol is alive and adapts itself to a culture and a time. Using symbols for complicated feelings was known to our primitive ancestors and to modern man. We find symbols in art, religion, politics, advertisements and in our daily lives. It is interesting to examine the history of these symbols to see if there is a relation between the new symbols and the old ones.

The central idea involved in searching for symbolic meaning is that a symbol consists of various elements and that there is a visible form and an invisible meaning. To understand the psychological meaning of symbols, we can draw on a number of sources since, in principle, everything in nature, the world and the universe can be used as a symbol.

1.4   The meaning of a symbol

If we want to discover the symbolic meaning of, for example, the bird, we would use the following approach. We start by studying the biological characteristics of the bird: what is a bird, how did it evolve, which sorts of birds are there, how and where do they live, what does it eat, how does it reproduce, how does it care for its young, how does it relate to other animals and how does it relate to humans? We would examine how birds have survived in nature, in captivity (a birdcage) or in a modern metropolis.

After having gathered sufficient information about the bird in all of its natural habitats, we would begin to search for the meaning of birds in human history and in mythology, sagas, legends, religions and Bible stories. Books in which symbols are explained often point us to these stories, as, for example, the *Herder Lexicon*, Hall's *Encyclopaedia*, Timmer's *From Anima to Zeus*, *The XYZ of Mythology*, *Who's who der Tiere*, *Worterbuch der symboliek*, etc.

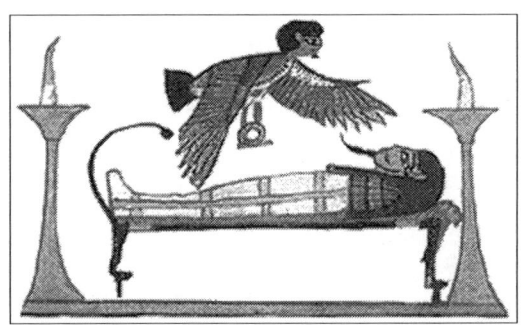

Ba (= bird=soul=breath) leaving the dead body.
From: The Egyptian Book of the Dead

In various cultures and in various periods, there are stories in which birds appear, and we can also find fairy tales in which a bird plays an important role (Grimm, Chinese, Russian, etc.). In M.L. von Franz's books, various motifs in fairy tales are described, and the psychological significance of figures in these fairy tales is explained. This is also investigated in books by *Verena Kast, Marian Woodman and Clarissa Pinkola Estes*; in the *Collected Works* of C.G. Jung, an index can be used to find indications of an archetypical meaning. Finally, we also must consider the personal meaning of a symbol. In this present example, that would involve studying the personal experiences that someone has (had) with a bird and the feelings that played a role. Only after we have examined as many aspects as possible of a symbol can we defend the symbolic meaning that we assign to it.

In this way, we can examine the meaning of symbols of people, animals, things, natural occurrences, etcetera. All of this shows how impossible it is to expect that there is a dictionary or a book of symbols that can be quickly consulted to find the meaning of a symbol in, for example, a child's drawing. However, books of symbols can be used to understand aspects of parts of a symbol. A symbol is complex in the sense that it can lead to many explanations, some of which contradict the others. For example, a vulture is greedy and waits until an animal has died so it can eat the body. But, on the other hand, a vulture is very useful because it eats dead meat so that the body does not fester or begin to stink. As this shows, it is not correct to put a value judgement on a symbol or to say that something is good or bad, negative or positive. What is so special about a symbol is that, although it can express polarities and contradictions, it also contains a certain harmony.

If we wish to understand the symbolic meaning of an animal, a person or a thing in a certain drawing or statue, we will have to try to delve further into the symbol. As explained above, symbols are natural expressions thought of by humans and open to examination. When assigning a specific meaning to a specific drawing, we should also consider the meaning of other symbols used in the same drawing to see if there is a relation between them. In this way, we can solve the puzzle piece by piece. Studying the use of symbols in human history can help us to better understand the meaning of symbols. Fortunately, many symbols have been saved on, for example, the walls of ancient temples and buildings and in paintings, pottery and ancient art.

1.5   Symbols in art and religions

From prehistoric times and long past the Middle Ages, many paintings and sculptures were used to convey moral and religious messages to people who could neither read nor write. Life was regulated by the Church, and there was no division between church and state. The artists of that time searched for ways of expressing human emotions. The paintings of Hieronymous Bosch(1450-1516) are filled with hidden symbolic (alchemistic) meaning, such as in his *Garden of Delights*, a painting that seems to express the madness of humanity and human existence. It is an example of an era in which the earthly characteristics of human beings were expressed. After the Middle Ages and the Renaissance, there was a growing trend to paint people and the natural landscape according to nature. That was not simply a desire to do something different, but was caused by artists wishing to express the (as yet) unconscious feelings of mankind. As human beings became increasingly conscious of themselves and their existence, they began to question their origins and the meaning of life. Scientific discoveries about the earth and the universe were made (Copernicus, Galileo) that were contradicted by the ruling authority at that time, the Church. Artists, however, could continue to manifest themselves by symbolically expressing a more natural existence. Nature became a symbol for human nature.

The meaning of the symbols of alchemy plays an important role in analytical psychology. The symbolic language of alchemists, known since the 3rd century A.D., became especially prominent in the early Middle

Ages. It was C.G. Jung who recognised the true meaning of the symbolic language and signs of alchemy and appreciated their value. He showed that the alchemists were not just a bunch of men searching for gold but that they were independent, philosophical and psychological thinkers (C.G. Jung, *Psychology and Alchemy*, 1953). The processes they described to change stones into gold was a process of the psyche that could effect changes in human personalities. In actuality, the development of the process of individuation involved the transformation of the Self. The alchemists called the Self an internal divine power that, in principle, exists in every person. These thoughts were considered heretical by the Church, who believed that God directed human actions from above. The study of alchemy is difficult and complicated and does not need to be treated in depth in the framework of this book. But it is important to note that, through the ages, both alchemists and artists, by using symbols in their drawings, paintings and etchings, on clay and on stone, in books and in their writings, expressed the most important questions about life that were related to psychological feelings.

Those individuals who made drawings in the Egyptian tombs did not refer to themselves as artists, nor did the Australian aboriginals with their dream paintings before Western tradesmen began to sell these paintings as art. They used their work to express feelings that were essential and universal. This need still exists because it is in the nature of the creative individual to give external shape to his or her inner psychic processes. Sculpture, music and dance all have their roots in prehistoric people and are still present in every culture. They are no longer just an expression of religious feelings, but they reflect the basic feelings of every person; people need to express themselves in these ancient forms of expression. Music, for example, still plays a large role in important events, both at parties and at funerals.

Visiting a museum, attending a concert or a play, visiting old cities, churches and temples, enjoying modern architecture and landscapes, dancing on special occasions (be it the polonaise or the opening waltz at a wedding) are universal human pleasures. People evidently feel better when they participate in these activities. Art touches our deepest feelings, and these feelings are universal.

The Impressionists of the 19th and 20th century were searching for a new way of expressing themselves that was less focused on surface appearances. People were becoming aware of deeper emotions, something which coincided with deeper knowledge of mathematics and physical sciences. At the same time, theories about a more deeply lying psychology began to arise. People were looking for new forms and images such as those found by innovative artists such as Picasso, Van Gogh, Paul Klee or Dali. It is often said that it is impossible to discuss art; this same is true of symbols and religion. The reason for this is that both spring from the same source, the human psyche, and especially from the unconscious psyche. The artist knows this. There is not a single artist who would claim that he or she have 'thought up' their art. It has nothing to do with religion if artists claim that they feel that they have created something that came from outside themselves. Great artists have an inner source of divine inspiration, which has been given to them by the gods. Artists in all periods use symbols that suit their times and their culture. New symbols are not thought of by the intellect but rather they are the expressions of the thoughts, desires and fears that people share and that can be given shape in the form of spontaneous creative expressions such as images, music or dance.

CHAPTER 2

THE PSYCHE AND THE ART OF DRAWING

2.1 The unconscious as a psychological phenomenon

Among the many things that have been said and written about the unconscious is that children still live in the unconscious. But what do we actually mean by the unconscious? Some people believe that unconscious is synonymous with accidental and toss it off lightly as a coincidence, as something with no deeper significance.

The unconscious is a modern psychological phenomenon that has been a subject of investigation since the early twentieth century. Sigmund Freud, one of the pioneers in this area of investigation, described the unconscious processes that play a role in the psychological life of the individual and in society. It was Freud who discovered the aggressive and sexual libidinal impulses that influence a person's thoughts and actions. Particularly important to Freud's theory was the significance that he attached to the Oedipal sexual development of the child, especially boys (Peter Gay, *Freud: a life for our times*.)

A special description of the unconscious is that given by C.G. Jung:
"*While the personal unconscious is made up essentially of contents which have at one time been conscious but which have disappeared from consciousness through having been forgotten or repressed, the contents of the collective unconscious have never been in consciousness , and therefore have never been individually acquired, but owe there existence exclusively to heredity. Whereas the personal unconscious consists for the most part of complexes, the content of the collective unconscious is made up essentially of archetypes.*' (C.G.. Jung: *The Archetypes and the Collective Unconscious*, Second Edition, p. 42)

Jung discovered that, in addition to the personal unconscious, there is also a collective unconscious that forms the basis for our psychological life and that is the same for every individual. According to this theory, we all share collective unconscious feelings that we have inherited from our ancestors, just as we inherited biological human traits. The material about the development of consciousness and the unconscious in humans is very complex. Although the field of analytical psychology is only a few decades old, the sources on which it draws when interpreting the deeper layers of our psyche are centuries old, complex and abundant.

In his *The Origins and History of Consciousness*, Erich Neumann made an extensive study of the development of consciousness in human beings. Neumann explains that the mythological stories show us that the individual's process of becoming conscious is similar to the development of consciousness in humans in general. In Neumann's *The Great Mother*, he describes the special relation between a child and his or her mother.

2.2 The meaning of the mother archetype

The term 'archetype' is found in Jungian analytical psychology. An archetype is a primordial image or concept that has a deeper, more universal significance than a symbol and that derives from the collective unconscious. An example of an archetype is the 'Great Mother', an archetype that plays an important role in a child's psychological development. We will later see how children give expression to these primordial feelings in their drawings. Before turning to this, however, some background information about the concept of the archetype is necessary.

In the history of mythology, fairy tales and religion, the same motifs with the same meanings can be found in all cultures and periods. According to Jung, these motifs and thoughts arise from the collective unconscious, the basic structure of human characteristics. They are primordial emotions and desires, physical and psychological patterns of behaviour, that are common to all human beings. An example of a well-known archetype is the 'divine marriage' or the 'fairy-tale marriage' that symbolizes the union of two lovers. Such emotions, told time and again in myths and fairy tales, concern the efforts to unite opposites. This means that the individual knows that, deep inside, there are opposing traits (and desires) and that these traits (and desires) must be joined in harmony. What is important is not that every man finds the ideal woman or that every woman finds her prince, but that every man has to find *his own* opposite, the inner woman (the anima) and that every woman has to find *her own* opposite, the inner man (the animus). Anima and animus both have positive and negative characteristics.

To put it more simply, one of humanity's tasks is to become conscious of the dualism of human beings and to unite this dualism in harmony. Images (figures or statues) have been created for the anima and the animus and are called archetypes. These concepts or figures continue to reappear in dreams, myths, old tales and modern television shows. Female traits (the anima) are found in the good fairy, the wise old woman, the innocent virgin and the good mother, but also in the wicked fairy, the witch and the temptress. Male characteristics (the animus) are found in the explorer, the discoverer, the caring father and the wise old man, but also in the devil, the tempter, the tyrant and the power-hungry.

There are more archetypes for all sorts of human characteristics. The archetype of the child includes innocence, spontaneity, naïveté and dependence; that of the old king includes power, control, protection and wisdom. The archetype of the Great Mother has been expressed in all periods and cultures in a wide variety of art, stories and rituals, ranging from the earliest depictions of goddesses on vases, in statues, fertility goddesses, the Madonna and statues of Maria to modern depictions of women in contemporary art (Moore, Picasso). There are depictions not only of the good mother, but also of the terrible mother in the form of goddesses that can be devouring, deadly or destructive (Kali, Coatlique, snake goddesses, etc.).

Our predecessors experienced the natural world in which they lived and on which they depended for their food and protection as a sort of mother, Mother Nature. They were familiar with the positive aspects as well as the negative aspects of nature, such as darkness, floods, droughts and dangerous animals. They experienced the world mythologically, that is, they imagined the world in archetypes, one of which was the Great Mother. A newborn infant also experiences these archetypal feelings of an all-encompassing Great Mother on which the infant is completely dependent.

The assumption that children repeat the psychological development of their ancestors means that the young child experiences the world mythologically. As is known from modern child psychology, there is a symbiotic relationship between the baby and the mother in the baby's first stage of life. In a mythological sense, this means that the child experiences the mother as Mother Nature, a natural surroundings that offers protection and food. This is the archetype of the Great Mother.

This archetype is not the personal, individual mother but rather the archetype of the mother; it encompasses both the good characteristics such as protection and food as well as the negative characteristics such as darkness, fear and complete dependency. Only at a later stage when a child's own ego and consciousness have been formed does he or she recognize their mother as a personality.

2.3   The child and mythology

It is especially as a result of Erich Neumann's insights that we can compare the evolutionary development of the human psyche with the psychological development of the child (*The Child; Structure and Dynamics of the Nascent Personality*). We can understand the psyche of the child if we are aware of the history of the human psyche, a history that we recognize in mythological stories and images.

When people became conscious of themselves (as individuals and responsible personalities), feelings of fear and loss were set free (Erich Fromm, *Fear for freedom*). Human beings were expelled from the childlike paradise of the unconscious and had to rely on their own inner strength. Both the discovery and denial of this individual inner strength with both the positive and negative aspects led to the formation of archetypes. The process of becoming conscious was able to take place by representing these archetypes as gods and goddesses in mythological stories, by performing rituals or by depicting the archetypes as material symbols (totems, masks, stones).

Mythological stories were not invented by people just to amuse one another or simply to pass the time. Rather, the stories represent psychological emotions, emotions that arose from the moment that people began to ask why they had been born, what the purpose of life was and what was the source of all life. These same themes can be found in the mythological stories and old religions in North and South America, in China, among the Eskimos, in Africa, Asia, Australia, Egypt, etc. Their basic structures are clearly identical since the stories are about universal emotions that are experienced by people naturally. The stories were not invented, but rather they were present in human beings before they could be expressed.

Neumann compares the process of humanity's (and the child's) becoming conscious with the stories of the creation of the world that are found in all cultures throughout the world and that are very similar to one another. The feeling and intuition that the world was created and that the cosmos was somehow structured has been present in humans from the moment the human psyche began to develop. The most common stories of the creation of the world say that chaos, darkness, unlimited space and eternity marked the beginning. Then something – often described as an island, an egg, a piece of land or an animal – appeared. Water was divided from land, light appeared in the darkness, the sun and the planets were created, the earth was inhabited by animals and then by people, etc.

There are mythological stories about the wars among the gods and between the gods and their children, about battles between dragons and heroes, about resurrection and death. Erich Neumann describes the various phases of mythological history in connection with the great world religions and compares this with the rituals and customs in older cultures and in modern times.

During the course of a child's psychological development, children (just like their ancestors) become aware of the fact that they have to become adults and that they will have to take care of themselves. Children distinguish between positive and negative experiences and emotions. They feel love and hate within themselves and in others. While becoming adults, children become aware of the fact that they are dependent on nature and that they are mortal. In the first years of life, young children experience the world just as their ancestors did, a world of which magical forces, monsters and dangers in which they need support and protection from others. Primitive people lived in fear of the sun's failing to rise each morning. They ascribed supernatural powers to animals, trees and celestial bodies. Even though we modern adults are aware of the laws of nature, quantum physics and the universe, we are still in awe of nature's enormity and unpredictability. The feeling of being dependent on something large and unknown is universal.

While growing up, every child experiences the inner tendency to become conscious of himself or herself and to discover an inner personal core. This is even true in young children when, at about the age of four, they begin to think independently and to ask questions about where they come from, where they were before they were born and where they will go after they die. Every individual has to discover who he or she really is and what the purpose of life is; every person has to search for the undiscoverable treasure. This is the road to individualization. Children set out on this road spontaneously, without being ordered to do so by others, just as their natural instincts tell them that they have to drink, sleep or walk.

The presence of old mythological stories in the modern world has been demonstrated by Joseph Campbell, a scholar generally considered to be the most important expert in the area of mythology. He states, for example, that the Oedipus figure, even today, is standing at the corner of the road waiting to cross (Campbell, *The Hero with the Thousand Faces*). Mythological stories represent important psychological emotions that have remained in all periods and cultures.

Old mythological stories are told and experienced again and again in the desires, reactions and emotions of people in this day and age. As an example of this, we can point to the worldwide reactions of mourning at the death of Lady Di, who could not marry her lover Dodi. Their untimely deaths resemble the legend of *Pyramus and Thysbe* as told by Ovid, or Shakespeare's *Romeo and Juliet*, or even the more modern musicals such as *West Side Story* and *Miss Saigon*. The fairy tale of two lovers who, despite strong protests, wish to marry represents the human desire for union and harmony between opposites. If this union and harmony is not achieved, the consequences are fatal for both sides (Marian Woodman wrote of this in *The Maiden King*).

Another modern myth is told in the *Harry Potter* series about a child who feels lonely and deserted and who goes in search of his true identity. His search can be compared to Jung's process of individualization. The archetypal child (the divine child) who has an inner desire to be found refers to the many mythological stories and fairy tales about a child who frees himself and who is saved by others in order to discover and show who he really is. This means that, even if a child (or an adult) has had no experience of adoption, neglect or abuse, there is still an inner desire to be found. The abused or neglected child is part of our own unknown and unused psyche that is hidden away in an unconscious, dark corner.

Primitive people were able to express these emotions artistically in drawing, music, dance, theatre and poetry. All peoples and cultures dance, make music, perform plays and carry out rituals. The art (the skill) to express these emotions, which has always been present in every individual, begins in childhood with games and drawings. For this reason, we can say that, when children begin to depict their surroundings and their emotions in symbols (as in games and drawings), they have begun to express their inner (mythological) emotions. Special circumstances can prevent children from following this natural tendency. They are psychologically tied so that no healthy development can take place. We can observe the psychological development of children by looking at their drawings, games and bodily movements. We can see if a child has difficulty in a certain phase of development and we can create circumstances in which children can freely express themselves in stories, fantasy figures and games, just as our ancestors did in their mythological stories, rituals and dances.

2.4 Body and psyche

The body plays an important role in how we express our emotions. We can trace the development of human physical characteristics back to the biological beginnings of our existence. Life on earth probably began with the formation of organic connections in the primeval atmosphere (oceans). According to the biological theory of evolution, this was followed by the formation of plants and (one-celled) animals. The beginnings of human life hold few mysteries for us. We are familiar with depictions of the egg and the sperm cell as well as of the human embryo in all of its stages. Lennart Nilsson's book *A Child is Born* contains magnificent photographs of these earliest developments. In the uterus, a group of cells is formed from which develops a snake-like/fish-like being. We can see a tiny person with a coccygeal vertebra and a large head that can move around in the uterus. The development of the spinal vertebra, lungs, eyes, ears and nervous system are displayed and described. We act, think and behave as humans and we 'know' even in the uterus that we are predestined to become a human being. A number of factors, including inherent factors, surroundings and experience, result in specific personal characteristics being formed. Personality is partly shaped by experiences and insights and this is a life-long process.

Research in evolutionary, biological, psychological and cultural development show that the child repeats the psychological prehistory of human beings just as the embryo repeats the biological development. It is generally recognized that the physical development of the human embryo shows similarities to the development of human beings. The fetus in the uterus repeats the biological development of its ancestors. This process does not end at birth. The baby is still completely dependent on the mother and the surroundings. After a few months, the baby beings to crawl and to explore and, some months later, the baby can stand and walk. But during the first year of life, the child cannot talk and has no consciousness. In the course of time, the child learns to see and recognize the things and people around him. He or she develops a unique personality that is aware of itself and is interested in the surroundings. Children first find themselves in the protective surroundings of the family, where they learn to develop intellectually. Having become an adult, they leave the family, set off in search of their own way and can finally fend for themselves in new surroundings.

During the course of millions of years, our ancestors experienced this same process of becoming conscious. In the beginning, there was an ape-like creature that was unaware of itself and dependent on Mother Nature for food and protection. It first moved on four feet and later evolved into a human that could walk upright. Humans further evolved in their use of language and their growing intellectual consciousness. New regions were explored and physical and mathematical laws were discovered. The cultural, social and industrial revolution helped to shape modern man. But only about 100 years ago were both psychology and psychiatry recognized as science and did we begin to become familiar with the psychological processes that come from our unconsciousness.

The development of a consciousness of the psyche cannot be separated from that of an awareness of the body. A person points to his body as 'himself' when he says 'I am'. The very first life experiences are experienced through the senses of touch, smell, taste, sight and hearing. It is especially these early experiences from the pre-verbal and pre-symbolic time that are stored in the body and in our physical knowledge.

In her book *Sand, Water, Silence, The Embodiment of Spirit,* Mary Jane Markell describes the inextricable connection between body and spirit that can be seen in a sandplay therapy process. Citing what Jung called the 'the participation mystique', she writes: *'We all have access to that instinctive animal wisdom through our mind-body being, the body-self, in which our every sound, gesture, silence or motion expresses itself through our senses, body, breath, and movements'* (page 204). Our bodies, brought into motion by our hands, can express pre-verbal experiences in dance and motion. The movements of our hands when working with material such as clay, wood, paint and pencils can give form to our early and non-verbal memories.

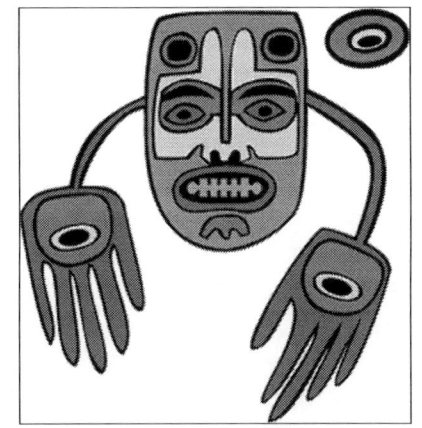

Kudush from a Modoc Indian legend (South America)

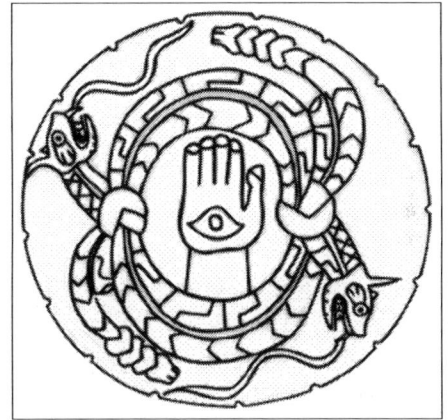

Ceremonial disc, rattlesnake/ eye in hand (Moundville, Alabama)

There are many old drawings that depict the combination of the eye and the hand. This shows that, ever since the earliest times, people have known there was a connection between eyes and hands. The eyes are the symbols of insight, the hands the symbols of creation.

Neurological research has shown that memories of images without titles can be recognized by the right half of the brain. This is the same hemisphere in which (unconscious) hand movements are executed, thus mirroring the Dutch saying 'When the mouth is silent, the hands talk'.

In spontaneous drawings and other artistic forms of expression, the hands express unconscious inner feelings. Dance therapy and psychomotor therapy make use of physical expressions of the entire body that come from the psychological unconsciousness and that reflect earlier physical experiences.

Creative individuals who are closely connected to their group and their culture will be the first to give expression to their emotions. As the history of drawing and art shows, ever since earlier times man has been able to express new, as yet unknown inner feelings in art.

2.5 Healing art

Expressing emotions has a positive influence on the human psyche. The term 'healing art' means that the process of healing is set in motion by the use of art, dance, music, theatre and storytelling. Therapists who use such creative means in their therapy have seen healing processes take place in their clients and patients. The healing effect of creative artistic processes on the psyche has been demonstrated by innumerable case studies and forms the basis of various theories on the effect of creative therapy, music therapy, dance therapy, art therapy, sandplay therapy, etc.

Few tangible expressions of art from earlier periods remain since many have been destroyed or lost. Stories and rituals were preserved in mythology and fairy tales that were passed from one generation to the next and were later recorded in writing by Homer, Virgil, the brothers Grimm, etc. The oldest human drawings that are still intact are the prehistoric cave drawings. The cave drawings in Lauscaux (southern France), thought to be about 17,000 years old, are the oldest known human drawings.

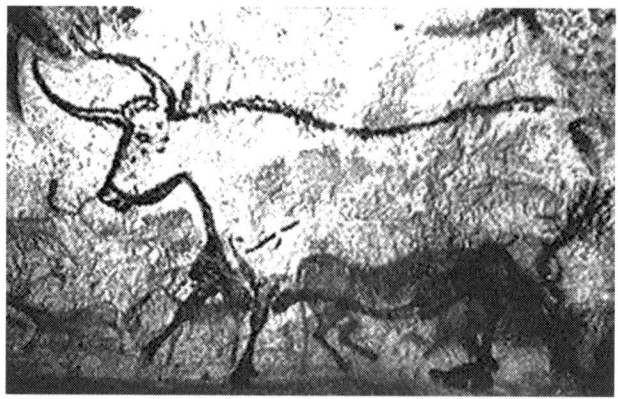

Cave drawing (Lauscaux, France)

Similar sorts of prehistoric drawings have been found in caves in South Africa, China and South America. People have been amazed by the technical quality of the drawings and have speculated about their meanings. The high level of technical quality suggests that people had been drawing for a long time and that even earlier drawings may some day be discovered. The cave drawings usually depict animals, hunting scenes and/or people in motion. The depictions have been studied by countless experts who have tried to understand their significance. Because the caves were difficult to reach and the roads leading to them were dangerous, the drawings are often almost intact. We assume that the roads to the caves were difficult in earlier times as well.

Erich Neumann gives a psychological meaning to these cave drawings by suggesting that prehistoric man walked the difficult roads to these caves as a sort of ritual and that they used the caves as temples. He further suggests that the walls and ceilings of the caves were decorated with drawings of the animals that had to be killed because prehistoric man was dependent on these animals (*The Great Mother*, page 8).

Working from this theory, we may assume that the drawings had a psychological meaning and were connected to such feelings as guilt and fear. We can also imagine that the group of hunters felt better on the return journey than on the way to the hunt. The meaning of going somewhere, being on a journey, is that a goal must be reached. The meaning of being on a journey, both in reality and as an inner experience, is still expressed in ritual journeys, processions and pilgrimages. This is also true of demonstrative marches in favour of or against something, since a demonstration is a collective message to the rest of the world that a group of people is on a journey to a collective goal. In earlier times and today, such a demonstrative march gives rise to feelings of collective strength, cooperation and a stronger personal peace of mind.

There is another factor that we can recognize in the proposed significance of the prehistoric cave drawings and one that plays a role in today's psychotherapy, namely, the healing effect of art as a means to express inner emotions.

As in prehistoric times, human signs are still deposited at places where someone has come for the first time, such as a mountain top, a deep cave or even on the moon: a name, a date or a cross. Writing and drawing on stones and walls has remained in force throughout the ages. They can be found in the Egyptian tombs (17th century BC), in special temples in Pompeii (80 AD) and in the Sistine Chapel in Rome (about 1500 AD). Some of these drawings have been saved simply by chance, such as those in tombs, pyramids and caves; others, less protected from the natural elements, have undoubtedly disappeared in the course of time.

A modern example of drawing on stones and walls is that of contemporary graffiti, which began in the 1950s and 1960s. Graffiti can be found in metro stations, on the walls of old buildings or under viaducts and bridges in the United States, China, Japan and throughout Europe. Could we say that this graffiti made by young people who congregate in the large cities at night to leave these illegal drawings has the same psychological background as the cave drawings? Is it just coincidence that graffiti came into being at the moment that the computer made its appearance and threatened humans with becoming just a number, of losing their identities? Graffiti began in the age of the hippies, the time of a new self-consciousness. Is it coincidence that at the moment when modern man began to consume his natural resources and thus destroy that on which he depended that groups of people began a journey to seek reconciliation with the gods? Young people in New York and, later, in other parts of the United States and Europe did not regard themselves as artists; rather, their graffiti sprang from an inner need, just as prehistoric artists made their cave drawings from an inner need.

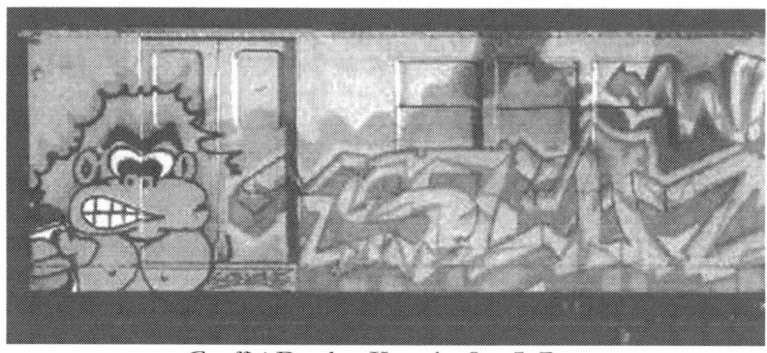

Graffiti Donkey Kong by Son I. Rem
(125th Street and Broadway #11RT Manhattan 1983 New York, USA)

The first modern graffiti was made in the underground (!) subway stations in New York City. In the beginning, one word, known as the 'tag', was drawn, and this was later expanded with more decorations and drawings. The first tags were probably used by street gangs to mark off their territories, but graffiti was also being used as a sign of protest against something happening in a city, a country or in politics. The image and the word are interwoven with each other in graffiti, something that can also be seen in the illustrated books made by the monks in the Middle Ages when a single letter, an initial, was decorated and thus received a special significance. The symbolic meaning of a letter in the alphabet can be found in the history of written language. According to the latest anthropological, biological and neurological research, this was the result of gestures and expressions of the face and hands.
The similarities between prehistoric cave drawings and graffiti are the rather inaccessible places they are found, the ritual journeys and the expression of inner feelings in drawings.

Graffiti still exists, although its psychological power of expression seems to have diminished now that governments have allocated places where graffiti is allowed. In fact, at places where, for example, a city council wants to have some decoration in the form of graffiti, there is little enthusiasm to provide it. The graffiti artist prefers difficult, forbidden, inaccessible or dangers locations.

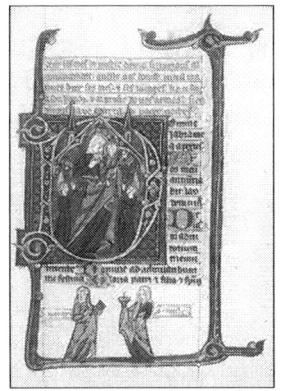

A decorated initial letter from a Book of Hours

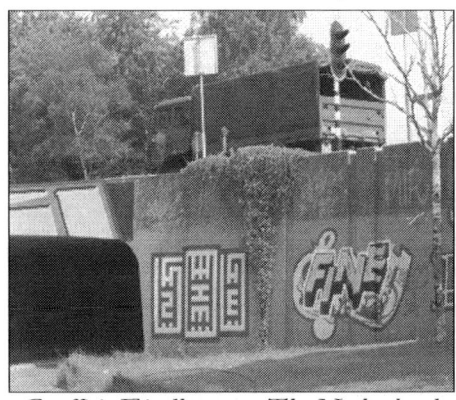

Graffiti Eindhoven – The Netherlands (2002)

Perhaps the digital highway and the Internet will again offer artists the chance to manifest themselves in secret. It seems that there are now 'silicon cartoons', microchips with molecularly small drawings (from twenty to two hundred thousandths of a millimeter) that have been placed there by chip designers using the plastic surgeon's micro-tools. Thirty-five of these designs are known, and it is thought that there are more designs that 'have not yet been seen by anyone' *(www.micro.magnet.fsu.edu/creatures/technical/packages.html)*.

These designs can be viewed only by using a very advanced digital microscope. Here again we see how humans adjust to the times and surroundings in which they live and find a way to decorate hidden places with their drawings and signs that have special significance and that most people (still) do not completely understand!

CHAPTER 3

DRAWING AND PSYCHOLOGY

3.1 Developmental psychology and the first years of childhood

Children draw in specific ways at certain ages, which is why it is necessary to refer to developmental psychology when looking at children's drawings. Since the beginning of the twentieth century, serious research has been done on the psychological development of children. This first focused on the area of intelligence (Binet). Even before World War II, and especially in period immediately thereafter (1945), a great deal of research was done on the effects of traumatic experiences on children and the consequences of theses experiences on the developing personality. Although there was much speculation, most researchers agreed that a traumatic youth could have many negative consequences for the adult. Sigmund Freud's daughter, Anna Freud, who had fled to England during the war, worked in a children's home and researched the problems experienced by evacuated children who had suddenly been separated from their parents. After having done further research on the development of children in special circumstances, she published two works on her findings: (*Normality and pathology in childhood, assessments of development* 1966).

In the 1950s and '60s, large research projects were initiated that still form the basis for many theories about the psychological development of children. The British psychoanalyst Margareth Mahler developed the separation-individuation theory, which she put forth in *The Psychological Birth of the Human Infant* (1957). This theory was very influential in how others viewed the psychological development of children between the ages of 0 and 4. Pioneers in the field, such as René Spitz and John Bowlby, observed the bond between mother and child and the importance of constant maternal care. Their findings resulted in more humane measures being adopted in children's homes and gave support to the view that it was better to have young hospitalized children cared for as much as possible by their own mothers. In this same period, Erik H. Erikson studied the significance of the family and cultural surroundings in relation to the child's development. Based on Erikson's studies, D.W. Winnicot developed a form of play therapy and discovered the importance of drawing and playing. Piaget described the child's cognitive development in his theory about the phases in the child's powers of observation and thought. Others, such as E. Fromm, studied the influences of culture and politics on the development of personality. Many other publications appeared in the area of educational science (Bühler, Van Andel, Spock, Bladergroen), especially written to help parents raise their children. These sorts of publications disappeared in the 1960s and '70s in the face of anti-authoritarian principles of childrearing when parents no longer wanted to be told how to raise a child. Further research representing different schools and theories continued to be published, sometimes supplementing and sometimes contradicting one another, but few new insights into child psychology were added.

Present-day child psychology still rests on the pillars of post-war theories, although our knowledge of cognitive, motorial and analytic areas has greatly expanded.

In the 1980s, Alice Miller received a great deal of attention with her books *The Drama of the Gifted Child* and *For Your Own Good*. In these books, Miller writes about 'poisonous pedagogy', a traumatic manner of childrearing that is denied by both the parents and the child and that damages the psyche of the child, who has to constantly adjust to new demands.

3.2 The separation-individuation theory

The discussion of the significance of children's drawings put forth in the following chapters is based on the well-known psychological theories of child development, especially those of Piaget, Winnicot and Mahler, who studied infancy and early childhood and the development and significance of games. In addition, evolutionary, symbolic and mythological explanations based on Jung's analytic theories and Neumann's theories of child development will also be used.

Because Margareth Mahler's separation-individuation theory plays such a large role in the first years of a child's life, it is useful to examine this theory more in depth. When a child is born and the umbilical cord has been cut, the child becomes an independent human being who can breathe, eat and perform all of the bodily functions that had previously been performed together with and dependent on the mother. Mahler calls this the 'biological birth'. After having been born, the child is still completely dependent and must be nurtured, kept warm and cared for to survive. Both prior to birth and several weeks (perhaps months) following, mother and child are in the so-called 'symbiotic phase', a phase in which mother and child are dependent on each other and in which they can sense each other's needs. Just as the mother knows that she can no longer keep the child in her womb, the child knows that he or she must be born. In the first few weeks or months after birth, this symbiotic relationship continues in the areas of feeding and care. The newborn infant is not capable of distinguishing his or her own body from the outside world. The child feels identical to the world: he or she is the world, powerful and egocentric.

Gradually, a division begins to form between the child and the outside world. The child discovers the difference between experiencing himself or herself and experiencing something else. For example, the child discovers that sucking his own thumb feels different than sucking on his mother's thumb. The child explores, compares and experiences *difference*. We assume that the symbiotic phase lasts for 6 weeks to 3 months. This not only varies with each child, but the transition to the next phase is a gradual one with regular regressions to earlier phases.

Mahler believes that a child is biologically independent when the umbilical cord is cut, but that the child is not psychologically independent until about his or her fourth year. She calls this independence the 'psychological birth'. Mahler explains that the symbiotic phase is first followed by a phase of *separation*, in which *individuation* can occur. A premature separation can cause a sense of having been abandoned because the psychological mechanism cannot yet deal with this feeling of separation. On the other hand, a possessive mother can obstruct the development of separation even though the child is prepared both bodily and cognitively. Separation means that the child feels himself to be an individual 'separated' from the mother, his 'own person'. This must not be confused with being 'separated from' the mother in the physical sense.

If separation proceeds well, the first phase of individuation can take place. In this earliest phase of self-identification, it is not a question of 'who I am' but rather 'that I am' (Mahler, page 8). According to Mahler, only at about the age of four does a child reach a certain psychological independence and can we speak of a 'psychological birth'. Mahler's studies and publications about infancy and early childhood, together with those of her contemporaries (Bowlby, Erikson), are even today very influential in underlining the significance of the mother-and-child relationship. The binding theory that developed from this is recognized by modern psychological researchers.

According to analytical theory, the primary relationship between the child and the mother (that is, between the child and the world) is the basis for subsequent relationships with the world outside. A safe primary relationship with the mother will enable the child to grow towards a safe relationship with another, with all of the adhering possibilities and developments. But if the basic relationship is damaged, the child will remain dependent and will be obstructed in his development. Such a damaged relationship can be repaired in therapy by making use of symbols. In an artistic and creative process, the child can again be brought into contact with an 'inner mother', the archetypal force that is present in every human being. Such a therapeutic process (in an adopted child) has been described by Andreina Navone, a Jungian analyst and sandplay therapist working in Rome. (*The Double Birth: A Clinical Story of Emanuele*) (Journal of Sandplay Therapy. Volume VII, number 1, 1998)

The physical, emotional and social development of babies and very young children is so fast and intense that, if it were to continue, every child would be a giant and a genius by the age of twelve. Fortunately, both physical and psychological growth are slower from the ages of about seven to twelve, a period known as the 'latent phase' (latent meaning hidden, invisible). The first four years of life are intense; a tremendous number of things happen and the child gains intense experiences. The child needs to deal somehow with these intense experiences and to still be capable of dealing with the following phase. The psyche has to be put to work, often through a process of repetition. We know that impressive experiences have to be told and experienced again and again in order to assimilate them.

Some people think it is an exaggeration to suggest that children need to deal with the first years of life, including pregnancy and birth. But they are mistaken. Although the delivery is a natural and inevitable process for both mother and child, it is usually a painful process. And especially nowadays, when many children are born with medical and technical assistance, the risk of a traumatic experience during and after the pregnancy and birth, such as an incubator or an operation, has become much greater. Growing from a child to an adult is also a natural and inevitable process that includes painful and frustrating situations for all of us. To survive, people have developed ways of dealing with these frustrations. The most natural way, and one practiced by adults when they were children, is by playing, which is why children should be encouraged in all sorts of expressive forms.

3.3 Psychological research on children's drawings

The area of children's drawings is a new subject of study in the field of psychology, simply because children's drawings were not saved in earlier times. We can assume that, even long ago, children drew, but only when paper became common (late 19th century) and children began to go to school could drawings be saved, studied and compared. Before this, children probably drew on slates, with a stick in the sand, on windows or on mirrors. Some children became artists, and we know that some of these did draw when they were young. Drawing was usually seen as a pastime or game. Only when people started to save and collect drawings (especially at school) did research arise that showed that children draw according to a certain line of development. The same scribbles, lines, figures, people and houses were everywhere evident.

A large study of drawings by pre-school children was published by Rhoda Kellogg. Since 1928, Kellogg had collected nearly half a million drawings made by children around the world. She studied the artistic development and classified the general forms that were common worldwide. In her *Analyzing Children's Art*, Kellogg describes the basic scribbles, the egg-shaped structures, the middle points, the sun with its rays (and faces), the development of drawing people, etc. Only incidentally did she speak of the emotional significance of a drawing. The urge to make a movement was a natural and necessary one in children and one that caused certain lines to appear on paper. The images prompted aesthetic feelings of beauty and harmony. Kellogg's book was a plea to allow children to draw spontaneously, without drawing lessons. The idea of letting children draw freely, both at school and in their leisure time, was quite new for that time.

It is understandable that little or no attention was first paid to the communicative and emotional significance of drawings because, at that time, very little was known about the theories of Freud and Jung and there was little research on the psychological and emotional development of babies and toddlers. Nevertheless, following this period, a number of studies used children's drawings as a diagnostic tool. For example, it was discovered that the more details drawn by a child at a certain age, the higher the child's intelligence. But, since the results were later not in agreement with other intelligence tests, the use of drawing tests to measure intelligence was abandoned. Objective evaluations based on a Rorschach test or a Draw-a-Person (D.A.P.) test proved impossible and failed to give a reliable indication of a child's emotional state. It was especially common in the 1950s and '60s to judge drawings and children's drawings on the basis of their emotional content, but this was often speculation lacking a sound basis or theoretical foundation.

Many contemporary psychological and educational studies focus on children's drawings, the way in which children draw, how and why they begin, when details are added, how a drawing develops, etc. (Cox, Meykens). Cognitive development receives most of the attention in these studies. In the development theories proposed by Liquet and Piaget, the drawings of very young children are considered to be a form of play and practice (Glyn, Thomas). Generally speaking, modern psychology still pays little or no attention to the emotional significance of children's drawings. This is understandable because most psychologists are calculating and measuring. Statistics has become an important part of the psychology curriculum, and a psychologist will not make a statement that cannot be supported by measurable and valid statistics or research findings. They follow the laws of mathematics: one plus one is two.

Emotions are difficult to express in statistics, as, for example, is evident in the test in which a child is asked to draw a 'nasty person' for example, someone who steals sweets and other things' (Cox, page 83). This assignment ignores the child's personal interpretation of 'someone who steals sweets and other things' because, at a certain age and faced with certain emotional problems, a child who, for example, does not get enough attention, will also steal sweets or other things himself. Such a test asks the child to project a 'nasty figure' onto someone else. The emotional significance of such a drawing assignment can be so ambivalent and complex for a child that the results cannot be scored objectively. Researchers were interested in whether a child would draw a nasty figure larger or smaller, but they found no significant indications. This is logical since the test does not measure the fact that almost every child has stolen a sweet now and again from the kitchen cupboard and that the naughty boy or girl is referred to as 'bad or nasty'. Interpreting the psychological and emotional elements in children's drawings must take into account factors that differ according to the child, personal character, life experience, cultural circumstances and age. And if we add to this the complex interpretation of symbolic meanings, we can see that a mathematical formula has not (yet) been found for this, as for many other aspects of the human psyche. But that does not mean that children's drawings lack emotional significance.

To understand a child, it is important to understand that feelings and intuitions are the first functions that children develop in attempting to feel at home in the world. Only later are the functions of thinking and observing called into use. Consequently, we must not view children's drawings only with our rational functions, such as thinking and observing, and count details or measure the points between lines and surfaces. Much will be lost if we ignore the background of the child's emotional life and the relation between the child and the subject of the drawing. We must and may use our feelings and intuitions. A feeling or intuition is often rejected by psychologists as if they are afraid of thinking intuitively, something they regard as unscientific or woolly. However, one of the greatest mathematical thinkers, Albert Einstein, pointed to the need for scientists to think philosophically and intuitively. In his *Ideas and Opinions*, Einstein emphasizes the importance of intuitive thinking in developing concepts at a higher level. We are certainly in good company! A good researcher may see something special and his intuition tells him that it is important. He thinks about what he has seen and draws certain conclusions. He has become aware of something. New discoveries often happen in this way. As we saw in the description of the history of consciousness discussed in the last chapter, man's thinking and feeling resulted from his observing and intuiting.

3.4 Playing and therapy

Most psychologists agree with the assumption that the basis of learning how to deal with frustrations can be found in childhood. For a child, playing is the best way of expressing and coping with frustrations and emotions. One aspect of playing is drawing. By playing, we do not mean a pastime or an imitation of adult behaviour but an expression of inner feelings in playing and creativity that is important for both children and adults. Adults can also turn to creative and artistic activities, museums, music, theatre, sport and games to give expression to their daily frustrations and problems.

The history of mankind shows us that children have always played. Moving, singing, dancing, playing competitive games and playing with objects representing the adult world are known in all periods and cultures. In the Louvre in Paris, there is a clay depiction of the game of knucklebones that dates from the 5th century BC. In a fresco in Pompeii, we can find a drawing of a girl writing (or drawing) with a stylus. A doll dating from the 3rd century BC with arms that can move has come down to us from Asia Minor. A toy wagon pulled by a horse from The Roman Empire (*A. Willemsen*: Romeins speelgoed, kinderen in een wereldrijk 2003) In the Renaissance, little girls were given dollhouses and little boys received tin soldiers. In later periods, industrial tools provided increasingly varied toys and the world in miniature for boys and girls.

Therapists were late in discovering and describing playing as a means of therapy. Freud regarded playing as a wishful fantasy or the urge to repeat. At the beginning of the 20th century in England, Melanie Klein began to discover the world of playing. She fortuitously discovered the therapeutic value of playing when, during a session in which she was unable to establish contact with a child, she offered the child a box of her own children's toys. The child spontaneously began to play, and Klein discovered that the child used two small dolls to represent himself and his friend (Klein, *The psycho-analysis of children*, 1937]). Following this, the significance of playing in the broadest sense received a place in the most modern theories of developmental psychology.

3.5 Drawing and therapy

A study of the deeper significance of children's drawings ultimately brings us to the psychotherapists who have worked with children and who have observed the therapeutic effect of drawing and other creative forms of expression. Children began to feel better when they were given the chance to draw. An important psychotherapist in this field was Susan Bach who, in 1952, published her first study of drawings by children who were seriously ill. For decades, she collected, studied and evaluated thousands of children's drawings. In *Life Paints His Own Span*, she gives impressive examples of the extent to which children who are ill are aware of their dangerous and hopeless situations. She includes examples of drawings with signals about the fears and desires of these children and she also shows that some of these drawings were to a certain extent predictive. Other well-known psychotherapists who have worked with sick children and who have collected, analyzed and wrote about their drawings are Kasper Kiepenheuer (*Was Kranke Kinder sagen wollen*), Elisabeth Kübler-Ross (*On Children and Death*) and Gregg Furth (*The Secret World of Drawing; healing through Art*).

Art therapists have long known that artistic expression has a therapeutic effect. In most European countries and in the rest of the world, a degree in Art Therapy is offered by many universities, where it is often a combination of psychology and art history. In the Netherlands, programmers for art and therapy often make use of such well-known theories as those stemming from the anthroposophic school, the creative therapy based on the creative process (Smitskamp), appeal analysis (Brom and Kliphuis) and communication by visualizing as play therapy (Hellendoorn et al). There are various theories about using drawings as diagnostic material, one of these being the *Diagnostic Drawing Series or D.D.S.* (Fowler and Cohen), which was recently introduced in the Netherlands. In England, the Dutch creative therapist Marijke Rutten-Saris received a degree for her research on drawing as a diagnostic instrument that included an analysis of movements made when drawing, known as the *Rutten-Saris index* (2002). We do not yet know the extent to which these tests will be recognized internationally, thus providing a breakthrough in appreciating the value of drawn material for diagnosis and treatment.

3.6 Jungian analytical therapy

Analytical psychology brings us to the deeper layers of the psyche and the meaning of symbols. Using this in addition to the theories and insights provided by sources such as modern developmental psychology, art history, anthropological and cultural anthropological research, and creative therapy, we can attempt to understand the significance of drawings.

Since the 1980s, Ingrid Riedel, a Swiss Jungian analyst, theologian and philosopher who is a professor at the Jung Institute in Zurich, has been publishing on the significance of drawing and painting in a therapeutic process. Among the subjects she writes about are the symbolic meaning of drawing and how drawing (and painting) can help people to face their problems and – more important – solve these problems themselves. The meaning of symbols with archetypal content and the collective unconscious are Jungian ideas and theories that are especially used in a non-verbal therapeutic process. In most European countries, the United States and Japan, the Jungian theories on the explanations of symbols and forms are well known.

3.7 Sandplay therapy

The philosophies and religions of the Far East, such as Zen Buddhism, have begun to influence Western psychology, and the word 'spirituality' is commonly used nowadays. An integration of Western and Eastern philosophies is gradually taking place. Creativity and play, both non-verbal expressions unobstructed by language and test material, bring us with their pure and spontaneous expressions from our childhood into contact with the original and deeper layers of the psyche.

Sandplay was developed in the 1970s and '80s by Dora Kalff, also a Jungian analyst, who had studied at the Zurich Institute and who knew Jung personally. She was introduced to World Technique, a test for children developed by Margareth Lowenfeld that makes use of sand and miniature figures, and in England she worked with Winnicot. Dora Kalff discovered and described the therapeutic effect on the psyche of playing with sand in her book *Sandplay, A Psychotherapeutic Approach to the Psyche*. She visited Japan and studied under the Zen teacher D.T. Suzuki. In Switzerland, together with Erich Neumann, she developed the therapy that she called 'sandplay', originally for children and later for adults. The

International Society for Sandplay Therapy (ISST) was established in 1989. Dora Kalff spent a great deal of time in Japan, where sandplay therapy is well suited to the philosophical world of modern Zen Buddhism. At the International Congress for Analytical Psychology (IAAP) in Los Angeles in 1995, the Jungian analyst Harriet Friedman gave a paper on sandplay. The Dutch Association of Sandplay Therapy (NVST) was established in 2003. The therapeutic effects of sandplay on children and adolescents are currently being studied in Germany. Sandplay continues to receive a great deal of international attention, and each year brings new publications with theoretical background and examples drawn from practice (Amatruda, Amman, Bradway, Carey, Markell, Steinhardt, Weinrib). The use of sand in old rituals the world over brings us back to earth, the natural element so long disregarded by our modern Western culture. Contact with nature's rudimentary elements, sand and water, is made with our hands. Via the hands, a connection is made between the inner world of the psyche and the outside world. In sandplay, this connection is visualized in a scene set in a sandtray in which just one or any number of hundreds of miniature figures, such as houses, trees, animals and people, can be used.

Three-dimensional images are made in a specially sized sandtray. These sand images can be compared with two-dimensional drawings. At the international congress of the ISST in Switzerland in 2001, Yvonne Pennington presented her research on the development of playing with sand, water and (fantasy) figures in children. The similarity with the developments in children's drawings was remarkable and confirmed the theory that children have a universal way of expressing themselves in playing as well as in their art.

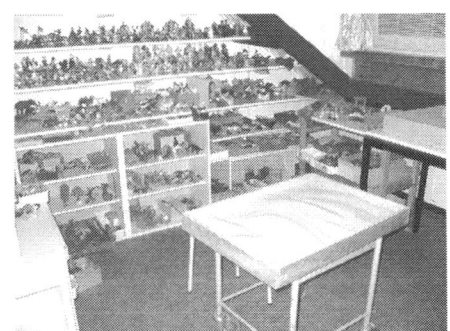

Sandtray and cupboard with miniature figures
Author's office, Nuenen, The Netherlands (2002)

CHAPTER 4

CHILDREN'S FIRST DRAWINGS

4.1 Universal drawings

Troughout the world and in all cultures, the first drawings that children make are always the same. So much research has been done on this that we can accept the accuracy of this claim.

Drawings can be signs that something is wrong but, before we can recognize these signs, we must understand the function and meaning of a normal drawing made by a child. In the same way, a physician must first learn how a healthy body grows and functions before he or she can spot abnormalities and illnesses. Only then can we look at the individual child and find signs of the personal development of the child's psyche in his or her drawings. The drawings reveal how and when the child has experienced a certain psychological phase of development.

Because the first children's drawings up until the age of four are an expression of the phase in which the child, according to Margareth Mahler's theory, has not yet been psychologically born, these drawings are so-called 'images of the past'. A child between the ages of two and four draws the period starting with conception. In their first years of life, boys and girls draw in exactly the same way. At about the age of four, the past has caught up to the present, and the child is able to further develop his or her unique personality. From this period onwards, we can see a greater difference in drawings by both boys and girls. We then follow the drawings done in the period up through puberty because universal psychological developments are still occurring in that period and we can recognize universal drawings up to that age.

Most children begin to draw at about the age of 18 months if they somehow get hold of a pencil. By then, the child can walk by himself and, although the child cannot fully speak, he or she understands almost everything others say. Children begin to repeat words they hear and, at the same time, they begin to draw. They begin to scribble and babble simultaneously.

The order in which the drawings described below are presented corresponds to the order in which children's drawings come into being. This is not a precise order because development and growth do not follow a mathematical curve. Rather, there is a back and forth movement in which different forms sometimes occur simultaneously or in which drawings at a higher level occur together with those at a more primitive level. The drawings may contain signals that parents should pay attention to. Because most parents are not used to looking at a child's drawing in detail, we will discuss the special characteristics of each drawing. Practice will help us to recognize the details in a drawing and to put aside the idea that the first drawings made by children are merely scribbles that do not represent anything. In fact, certain forms can be recognized in these early scribbles if we examine them well.

4.2   The drawing without borders

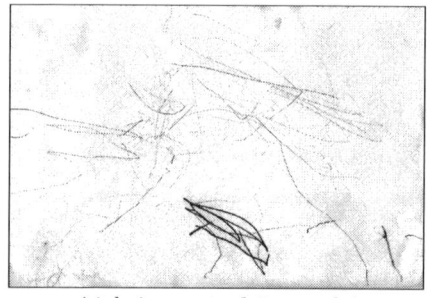 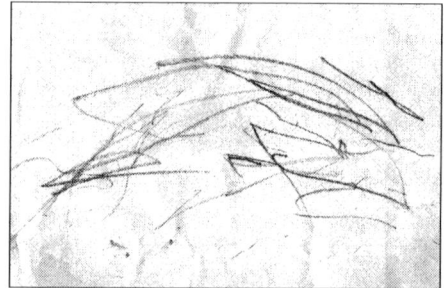

(girl, 1 year and 9 months)   *(boy, 2 years and 10 months)*

Description
*The drawing goes **beyond** the edges of the paper. The lines in the drawing go back and forth at random and in all directions.*

Significance
The first scribbles made by toddlers are all the same. The child's locomotion is not refined, movements are clumsy and holding a pencil is difficult. The lines go in all directions and no attention is paid to the edges of the paper. Although the child is not really drawing, the fact that 'something appears on paper' seems to be the most important result.

We can view these drawings made by children between the ages of one and a half to three years old as a physical expression of the feeling of boundlessness. The lines in these drawings resemble the movements made and felt by the embryo in the womb as it was rocked back and forth and moved at random in all directions. The unborn child, the embryo, does not know the limits of the womb in his or her earliest phase of development (until about 3 months after conception) and experiences boundlessness and unconsciousness.

Mythologically speaking, this can be compared to the period before the world was created, the phase in which chaos, darkness and infinity held sway. This is the prehistoric status of 'something being present' but not in time, only a status of infinity. There is no division between up and down, between heaven and earth. There are no contradictions. The questions of 'why' and 'from where' have not yet been asked. There is no sense of space and time.

The expression of the 'oceanic feeling' was first used by Sandor Ferenczi, a contemporary of Freud, and it is an apt description of the beginning of life. This oceanic feeling refers to the biological beginnings of our existence as primordial cells in primordial waters and can be compared to the egg in the amniotic fluid of the womb, fluid that is in many ways similar to the waters of the oceans in its salt and mineral content.

Some children suffered traumatic experiences, such as illness, infections or viruses, in the womb. Physical or neurological abnormalities that occurred in this prenatal phase can result in delayed development. Children with such abnormalities may continue to draw (and play) on the theme of boundlessness. If children continue to make these drawings of boundlessness even though they are no longer toddlers, we may wonder if there is some physical problem (i.e. spastic) or if there is a lag in development. But, from a psychological or physical point of view, these expressions of chaos and boundlessness may also be reactions to recent difficult or traumatic experiences.

Case illustration
A seven-year old girl came to my office. Her mother said that the girl was very active, did not listen to her parents and had difficulty sleeping. The parents had argued a great deal and had divorced a few months earlier. The father had moved elsewhere and had a new girlfriend who was expecting his baby.

When she came for the first time, the girl asked me if I had all of the colours of paint for her. She stood before the easel on which there was a sheet of paper attached to a sheet of wood. Using a brush and large strokes, she painted the entire paper; in fact, it seemed as if she did not see the edges of the paper because she also painted the wood to which the paper was attached! In the sandtray that was placed on a table, she scratched about in the sand with both hands, threw sand into the air and onto the ground, poured water from a watering can onto the sand, shovelled some sand into a bottle and then left everything lying as it was. She then went to the dollhouse where she played with the doors by opening and shutting them. Then she came to me and asked to sit on my lap. 'May I paint your face?' she asked.

Feelings of boundlessness, chaos and infinity are normal reactions to a traumatic experience. When hearing bad or disappointing news, 'the ground drops from beneath us', leaving us with no sense of time and space. It seems as if body and soul are roaming without purpose. Such feelings and experiences can happen to everyone. It is important that this phase passes and that a new phase begins, a new phase with more stability that can be expressed in drawings, play or behaviour.

4.3 The egg-shaped drawing

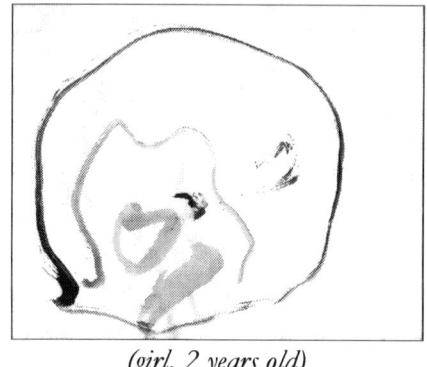 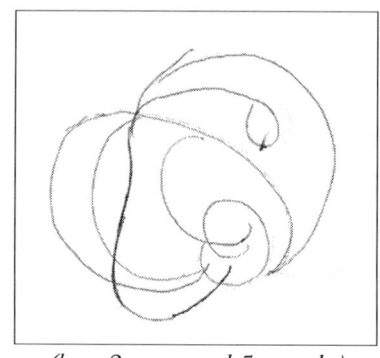

(girl, 2 years old)   *(boy, 2 years and 5 months)*

Description
An egg-shaped drawing in which at least one nucleus can be found. Drawings no longer go beyond the edges of the paper.

Significance
Compared with the boundless drawings that spill over the edges of the paper, a clear form can be recognized here. A number of forms are possible because of the variety in material and colour, but the egg-shaped form is the most recognizable. This is indeed a new form that can be drawn by children ranging in age from one and a half to three.

This egg-shaped form resembles the contours of the womb and contains a nucleus resembling an embryo or foetus. The drawing expresses feelings of security, of being the core or a part of something larger and of feeling protected. The experience without form or direction is followed by the experience of limitations and form. These are prenatal feelings connected to the time at which man became conscious of 'something' existing. Children make this drawing of an egg in just one movement. If children draw a lot, we see the nucleus in the drawing becoming larger and larger and gradually filling the entire womb. This phase is characterized by growth, and it is a joy to watch this process being drawn by healthy children.

The egg is both the beginning of something that is growing and the result of something that already exists. The feeling that the egg shape is related to the source of our existence can also be seen in the many mythological stories of creation told by various cultures. Many of these stories involve the 'round beginning', the nucleus, from which the world was formed; this is also known as the philosophical World Egg. There is also often mention of 'something' that was unknown and wants to make itself known. This 'something' is of divine origin. In symbolic language, the creation of the world is told as a division between land and water as if an island arose in the sea.

Sceptical readers may wonder how anyone can remember anything before their birth. It is possible that this memory is not an intellectual one but rather a physical one at an unconscious level. In his book *The holotropic Mind* Stanislav Grof, a well-known researcher in transpersonal psychology, describes the influence of the process of birth on an individual's later life. Current medical and biological research has also shown that the physical union between the mother and the unborn child leads to a psychological interaction between both. Both the mother's positive and negative feelings about the child can cause a reaction in the child.

In addition, there have recently been increasingly more indications of prenatal memories. It has been shown that a baby can hear his or her mother's voice when in the womb and can later recognize it, that they are accustomed to the barking of a dog, that they recognize and respond to certain pieces of music. The child responds to external circumstances beyond the womb and to internal chemical processes such as the use of medicine, alcohol or cigarettes. Emotional thoughts also cause chemical (physical) reactions in the body. For example, a pregnant woman is walking with her partner in the city and sees a couple with a baby carriage. Her partner remarks that they too will soon be walking like that. The resulting feeling (happy, ambivalent, tense) causes a physical, chemical reaction, such as feeling warm or cold, shivering or having an irregular heartbeat, that is similar to the butterflies in your stomach when you are in love. The heart beats faster, the blood flows more quickly. Chemical processes can be caused by the psyche. Feelings of fear cause an extra spurt of adrenaline. You do not have to take a pill to cause chemical processes to occur in the body. Consequently, we can assume that a baby in the womb notices 'something' and stores these observations in the body and the psyche.

The egg-shaped drawing is normal for children between the ages of two and three. The child has assimilated the boundless experience and has found a certain protection. A child draws this after the chaotic, boundless phase, and the drawing indicates a positive development. The child becomes aware of 'something'. The drawing also expresses the search for a middle point during that wandering in the watery phase of life. In addition, by making such a drawing, the child has created a certain protection for himself. If such an egg-shaped drawing is made when the child is a pre-schooler or older, it may be that the child feels uncertain. It may also mean that the child longs for security and protection.

Case illustration
When a five-year-old boy began therapy because he was having problems sleeping, he often drew these egg-shaped forms in the first sessions. He used felt markers for small drawings and paint for larger ones; he also made an egg-shaped house from clay. There were problems at home because the mother had gone on holiday by herself in order to think about her future relationship with her partner. The boy was quiet and did not want to talk with his father or other people. He seemed uninterested in the situation.

But with the egg-shaped drawings, he expressed his desire for security and created a safe place for himself. After this, the boy was able to tell his parents how and why he felt so sad and what he was afraid of. What he first expressed in symbolic language could later be expressed in words.

4.4 The snake-like drawing

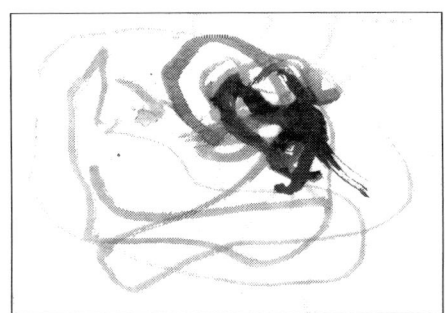
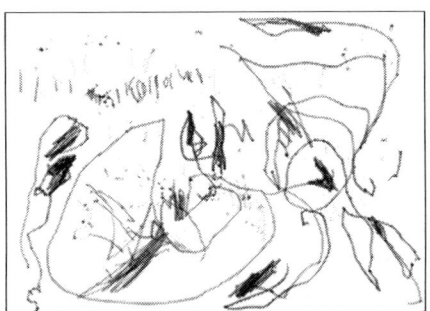

(girl, 2 years and 4 months)   *(boy, 2 years and 7 months)*

Description
There are long lines that are fish-like or snake-like. Sometimes, there is even a head and a tail.

Significance
As described earlier, the child repeats the biological developments of his or her ancestors during pregnancy. In the earliest stage, the embryo is a fish-like or snake-like creature, and a then more human form gradually takes shape. While swimming in the womb, the tiny person grows each day and notices the limits of the stomach wall. We can speak here of growth and movement.

The snake-like, slippery movements and the sloping lines can be compared to wandering through the earthly paradise. The snake has not yet appeared in its perfected form of the circle. The childlike psyche 'swims' around, unconscious of itself. This psyche is no longer just embryonic but is somewhat aware of itself; it lives in the all-encompassing container but gradually begins to become itself. The snake is a positive sign that mythologically means that man has been 'tempted' towards awareness. Freed from the unconscious state, man can begin to differentiate between above and below and to journey forth in search of a goal. The snake will eventually bite its own tail and form a circle.

Case illustration
During a lecture at the pre-school, a mother showed me a drawing made by her five-year-old son. She said that he could draw people but that, of late, he had been drawing watery lines that the mother could not interpret. When I questioned her further, it appeared that her son had been having trouble eating and had been acting like a child (wanted to be carried, cried at the drop of a hat, etc.). He had a one-year-old brother who had just learned to walk and who was making any number of discoveries so that the mother had to keep a constant watch over him. I told the mother that I thought the drawing showed that her son felt insecure. He would perhaps rather be small so that he could get more attention. I advised the mother to praise the boy for being so big and to ask the father to spend some time alone with him.

We examine the snake-like drawing made by this older child to see if the snake is swimming around without a purpose. Does the child have doubts about going on to the next phase or is he lazy? If life demands that a child make many adjustments, it is sometimes good to let the child 'swim'. We can see if this takes too long or if growth has halted or gone backwards. Nearly all children experienced the prenatal phase as one of happiness and safety. Feelings of unity, solidarity and joy are evidently feelings that cannot be experienced later in life. Some say that sex between a man and a woman and the climax of an orgasm are similar to the feelings of bliss experienced in the womb and that, because of this, sex is one of man's basic needs. Freudian theory says that man wishes to return to the status of the unborn child and its unity with the mother's body but that this desire conflicts with the natural desire of man to free himself of his unconscious state, to become independent and to differentiate himself from other similar creatures.

4.5 The spiral drawing

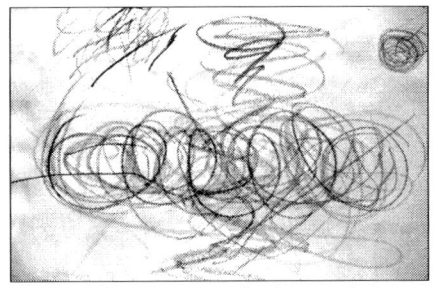
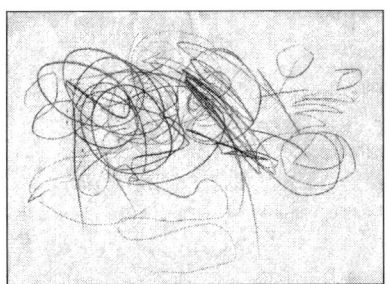

(girl, 2 years and 10 months)   *(boy, 3 years and 4 months)*

Description
In these drawings we can see large and small spiral lines. The spirals are drawn in one continuous movement.

Significance
Here we can clearly see a new form, the spiral, which can be recognized in drawings made between the ages of two and four. The form points to developing and unfolding, just as a new leaf on a tree unfurls itself. We can imagine that the spiral expresses the process of birth. During birth, there is a moment in which the baby is held fast, followed by a moment of release and development. Physically, the lungs unfold so that the baby can breathe independently after having uncurled itself.

It is remarkable how often the spiral is used in artistic expressions of life and death. In *The Tree of Life* by Gustav Klimt, for example, in M.C. Escher's *Vortexes*, or in the spiral designs on the Neolithic passage tombs in Newgrange, Ireland. The spiral form can also been seen in the development of DNA, the source of our existence.

Mythologically speaking, the spiral signifies finding a way out of unconsciousness, from passive to active, from maternal (material) to paternal (order), from analogue to digital. This differentiation in consciousness is expressed in such mythological stories as the struggle between the twin brothers Cain and Abel, the Egyptian Osiris and Isis and the split between the primordial parents. Moreover, the spiral is the first form in which time is expressed: there is a beginning and an end, distance and movement.

The spiral is a positive development in drawing and indicates a positive development in the child. As already said, these drawings repeat previous psychological and physical experiences; the child has found a way of giving external form to internal experiences. Finding a way out is one of the most important experiences of our lives. Repetition allows us to assimilate the experience, which explains why every child draws the spiral. Our biological birth is the first development towards and the first experience of a transition from darkness to light.

Children who draw spirals and adults who do this spontaneously or unconsciously (while telephoning, for example) express the fact that they have freed themselves from a situation or that they wish to do so. The spiral form can always be found in a phase of life that involves change. The child experiences a phase of struggle (clinging, afraid and stubborn) at about the age of nine months when he or she has to leave the symbiotic unity with the mother and become more independent. Adolescents can experience this same phase as they approach the phase of adulthood. And adults can also feel the need to draw spirals as expressions of ambivalence or the struggle to find a way out. The older child or the adult who draws many spirals may be expressing the wish to find a way out of a problem.

4.6 Children who do not draw

There are parents who claim that their child never draws. Because this may be caused by a number of reasons, it is good to know that children almost always express themselves creatively in one way or another, be it in games, music, dance or with toys. Drawings are not the only channel by which children express and assimilate the history of their coming into being. Some children 'draw' with their bodies or with toys. We can watch a toddler playing with a toy that goes every which way until the child begins to steer the car back and forth or in a circle. Or watch a child endlessly swinging back and forth on a swing. We can recognize boundlessness or spirals in many forms of play. Children do not draw only on paper but also in sand in a sandbox, on a window or on a door. And when they work with clay, these same forms can be seen.

There are also children who express themselves with their bodies. They sit in a toy car and drive around in it or they run in a spiral to the middle of a playground where they stand still. Certain ways of walking, running, dancing and making music can express universal forms. These universal forms, such as spirals, crosses and circles, also appear in traditional children's games such as chutes and ladders, tic-tac-toe and battleships.

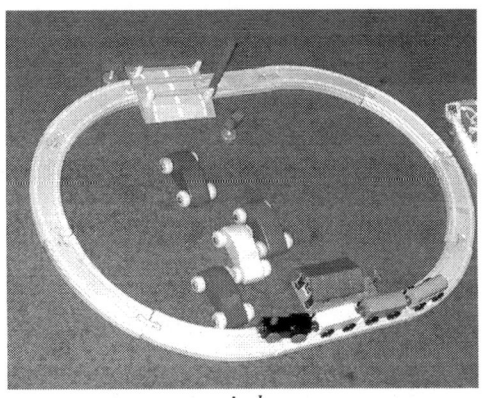
circle

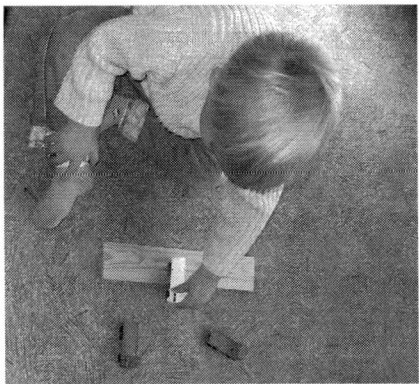
crossing

When playing, children make movements with their hand or entire bodies, and these are primordial forms and movements that can be found in all cultures. These universal forms that are expressed in rituals, games, drawing, painting, working with clay, dance and music are also the well-known components of creative therapy, such as art therapy, music therapy, or dance, drama or play therapies. Physical expression causes psychological processes to be experience and activated. This is also true the other way around: giving form to the psychological content causes physical activity and influences behaviour. This shows once again that physical and psychological developments influence each other.

4.7 Ego-consciousness and the Self

Ego-consciousness, that is, becoming aware of one's self, is an important basis for forming the personality, the development of which is present in every individual. Terms such as the Self, the ego, individuality, personality, the I, the conscious, the unconscious, the subconscious and I-awareness come from various psychological, psychoanalytical and Jungian analytical theories, and their meanings have been described in many different ways. Jungian analytical theory places special significance on the following terms: the unconscious, archetype, symbols and the

Self. The first three have been discussed in chapter one of this book. Those who wish more extensive information about Jungian theories can, of course, read Jung's *Collected Works*. Also of interest is M.L. von Franz's book *C.G. Jung. His Myth in Our Time*, a biography of Jung in which the author highlights his ideas and theories.

The Self is a typical Jungian expression. Jung defined the Self as having the psychological content of both the personal and the collective consciousness and unconsciousness as well as archetypal and divine images. It is that which makes an individual personally unique and generally human.

The search for the Self is the subject of many mythological stories. It is the treasure, the impossible goal, the answer to the question that the mythological hero strives for (King Arthur, Gilgamesh). It is the regulating centre that creates a continuous development and ripening of the personality. It is that which is inside each individual and which each individual searches for and hopes to attain throughout his or her life. There are contemporary mythological stories of heroes, such *as Lord of the Rings* and *Harry Potter*, in which the hero goes in search of 'that which cannot be said'. The circle (a ring, something round) is the perfect expression of the Self. Only after the Self has been made manifest can a truly unique personality be formed. This is a life-long process in terms of becoming conscious, self-realization, individualization, etc. This Self, as expressed in a circle and the mandala, has an archetypal significance. Finding the form of the circle is both the cause and the result of the growth of the Self.

Becoming aware of one's own body is the first step in becoming conscious of an inner (psychological) centre. This is followed by a phase of action and desire. The child, similar to his ancestors, is no longer driven by his temper or instincts but by 'I want'. An individual's will continues to develop throughout his or her life. In the primary phase, from before birth until several weeks thereafter, there is a symbiotic relationship between the baby and the mother in which the child feels physically and psychologically one with the mother. In the first few weeks after birth, a baby feels, tastes and smells no difference between himself and others. The child has not separated himself from the external world and is not yet aware of his own psyche. This stage is also called the vegetative or passive stage. The Self of the mother is still a bound to the Self of the child.

Psychopaths operate emotionally from the symbiotic phase. They are unaware of the difference between their feelings and those of someone else and, if involved in any violent action, they rarely feel sympathy for their victims. They cannot be blamed for this because they truly do not have knowledge of that emotion. They are usually not sentenced to prison but sent to a psychiatric institute for compulsory treatment.

This 'insensitiveness' is the feeling of a baby, focused on itself and familiar only with its own needs that, if not immediately satisfied, will lead to crying and screaming until someone comes. This behaviour is tolerated in a baby, who is gradually helped by sensible and caring parents to cope with such needs and desires as eating, washing, caressing and being loved. Children can postpone having their needs satisfied only if they know that they will be satisfied eventually. The rhythmical give and take between parent/guardian and child gives rise to the certainty that there is always someone who cares about you. In the first few months after birth, this give and take fills a mutual need. The mother's wish to give care causes the child to develop the need to be cared for. If the mother or guardian is ambivalent (for example, someone who is uncertain about whether or not the child is wanted or who doubts their ability to provide care), it will be more difficult for the child to develop his or her desires. An insecure child constantly whines and screams. Children who are neglected or abused never develop a sense of trust towards their parents or the world around them and can develop a psychopathic pattern of behaviour, such as an attachment disorder or a borderline personality disorder.

It should be pointed out that the term 'mother' does not mean the biological mother but rather the emotional, natural, caring and protective force needed by every child, that is, the so-called 'archetypal mother'. This security can be given by a parent or by any other permanent care provider. The most important factor is an unconditional, loving, regular and understanding relationship between the care provider and the child.

Between the ages of two and a half and three and a half, children develop a certain form of I-awareness. As already said, the core of the Self is present in every individual. The first possibility of activating the

Self occurs immediately after the symbiotic phase when the child of about three months old first senses separation from the mother (Mahler's 'separation phase'). This feeling is confirmed in the course of the next few months. We shall see below how important finding this core is to the further development of personality. We can see this in drawings with a circular form. A circle with a core. The child that finds the circle himself has found himself.

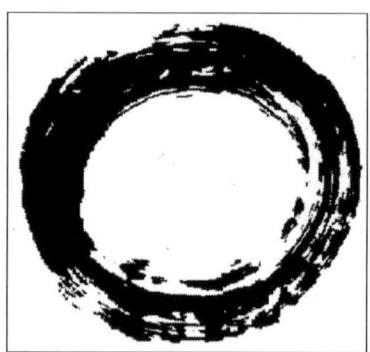

4.8. The circle

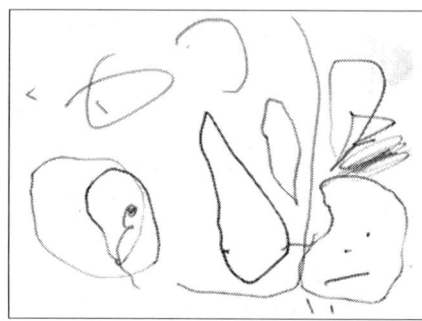
(girl, 2 years and 9 months)

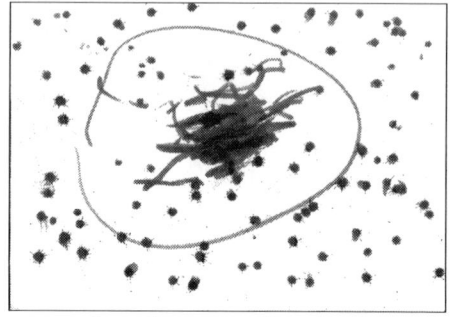
(boy, 3 years and 4 months)

Description
Left: various attempts at drawing a circle. Right: a circle with a core and dots inside and outside the circle.

Significance
The circle is important from a number of perspectives. The child's locomotion must be developed enough so that he or she can hold a pencil and draw a round line that closes. Cognitively speaking, the child needs to be able to estimate the space needed to make a circle. Drawings of spirals, which point to a certain physical and emotional development, are followed by the most important psychological phase: the feeling of one's own unique personality.

At this moment, the child discovers 'I am someone'. He or she simultaneously realizes that 'You are there too', that there is 'someone else'. The child discovers the borders between himself and his surroundings. He has also discovered that there is an emotional difference between what he wants and what the mother (or the external world) wants. The child discovers his or her own will. A baby or toddler's sense of I-awareness is first a physical feeling of a difference between himself and others. This primitive physical awareness is the basis that will lead to a deeper psychological Self that will continue to develop throughout the rest of the individual's life.

Between the ages of two and three, children begin to make circle drawings. In these drawings, the first awareness of a Self (at a deeper level) and an Ego (at a superficial level) are expressed in dots and objects that are found inside of the circle. Simultaneously, there is also an awareness of the other, so that something is drawn outside of the circle. This means that there is a sense of an inside world (inner) and an external world (behaviour). A child can then say, 'I *feel* unhappy and that is why I am crying'.

Case illustration
M. was a seven-year-old girl. As a three-month-old baby, she went to a children's day care centre for five days a week and later to an after-school programme. Her mother was ill and was often unable to give the child much attention in the first few years. She began therapy because she was very insecure, afraid and unable to defend herself. In the first hour, she filled ten sheets of paper (50 cm × 70 cm) with her paintings and was delighted that the entire office was decorated with drawings of bears, flowers, ducks, etc. She placed so many miniature figures in the sandtray that the sand was almost completely covered. After an hour, she skipped off and left me with the mess. I could conclude that she certainly had energy and creativity. At the next session, she

began by drawing faces and she sang a song about a circle with two circles, a nose and a mouth that she had learned at the day care centre. And she again drew the bears and the flowers. She evidently drew as she had been taught. She said that she could not draw something she herself had made up. The drawings had been taught to her and filled her need for control. But not expressing her feelings was at the expense of her sense of self-consciousness. Drawings that have been learned by the intellect represent a superficial filling in of personality, which does not lead to a feeling of oneness, completeness and uniqueness. When she finally began to draw spontaneously, she did so at a level that was too childish for her age; for example, she made drawings without boundaries, drew spirals and drew everything all together. In her therapeutic process, she came into contact with the neglected child. She felt small and abandoned and she expressed her fear and anger in play. By finally making a house of clay with a bed and a baby wrapped in a blanket, she created a safe place for the abandoned child. Following this, she turned to the archetypal 'good mother' when she put a motherly figure with a pram and a Madonna and child in the sandtray. We played store (giving and taking) and doctor (protecting and caring for).

One day when playing in the sandtray, she put a figure in each of the four corners. In the middle, she built an island and put a flamingo on top. She had found a centre and, as a result, herself. From that time onwards, her personality and her resulting feeling of security began to grow.

The circle or the ring symbolises both being shut out and belonging, both of which are important social experiences. A child can feel safe in a ring. In any number of games, a child can express the fact of having found a circle. For example, a child plays with a toy car that drives in circles around a middle point. Or toy cars (or other objects) are placed in a circle with something in the middle (a garage, a doll). A child plays, runs or dances in a ring. And a child enjoys sitting in a circle with other children and telling things. Someone can be the middle point of a closed circle. Things are different outside of the circle where things can happen that you cannot see because they take place outside of the circle. A child feels whether or not he or she has been included in or excluded from the ring.

If children do not draw a circle, we investigate whether or not they can play in a ring, whether they want to belong or prefer to remain on the sidelines. Can a child play a role in a ring and can he or she bear to be excluded (temporarily)? These are important social experiences that point to the universal human need to belong. This need is related to the development of the Self. The feeling of being a unique person can give rise to a feeling of loneliness and the need to make contact with another person. The basis for certain social skills is laid here.

Of course, a physical handicap can be the reason why a child cannot draw a (good) circle. In such cases, a healthy Self has been formed but its expression is hindered by, for example, a spastic handicap or neurological disorders. It is it important to pay attention to this because such a handicapped child could function well in a ring or place an object in its middle as in a sandtray.

Many adults are still searching for these basic feelings of the Self (and can still come into contact with them). 'I'm looking for myself' is an expression that many adults use in a certain phase of their lives if they go through an identity crisis. An aberration in the development of the unique ego-consciousness has consequences for the relations with others. People who are naturally themselves can accept the personalities of others. The Bible expression 'love thy neighbour as thyself' means that individuals must first become aware of themselves and must be capable of loving themselves before they can accept and love someone else as another person with his or her own Self. The inner feeling of oneness gives a child a basic feeling of certainty for practically the rest of his life.

4.9 Sunrays

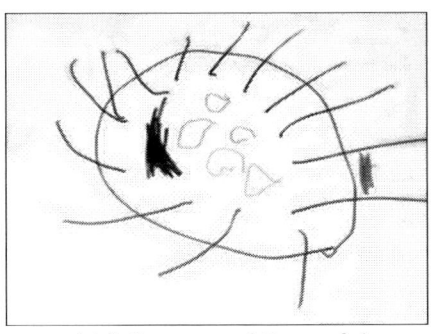

(girl, 3 years and 7 months)

Description
A circle with stripes that are drawn through the circle's edge.

Significance
This drawing usually comes after the circle, but they often occur together. The sunray drawing is a predecessor to the drawn sun. A three-year-old toddler does not usually give the name or meaning of sun to this drawing; it could equally be called a doll, a spider or a balloon. But if we look at the drawing, it seems to most resemble a sun, sometimes having something of a face. This is a universal form that appears in all children's drawings. In her book *Was Kinderbildern uns erzählen (1999)* Rose Fleck calls these rays 'feelers': from a point in the middle, the child is feeling the surroundings.

According to the previously mentioned separation-individuation theory of M. Mahler, the child begins to explore the external world after the individuation phase. In this drawing, we can see the attempts at separation in the rays that extend from the middle point of the circle. The child separates himself from the mother and dares for the first time to explore the outside world. The first attempts at separation occur at about the age of nine months and develop further as the child becomes physically more capable of leaving the mother (crawling and walking).

The child leaves the mother but wants to remain in her range of vision. He or she wants to be seen and wants to see the mother as well. This means that the child's exploration of the world occurs from a safe middle point. As already described in chapter 1 of this book, the child cannot remember that the mother is still present if the child cannot see her (Piaget's constant object). At this phase, the child is physically and psychologically dependent on and strongly tied to the mother or the permanent care provider. The child explores the world while remaining in contact with the mother. The sunray drawing is usually done after the child's third year, after the circle drawing, and is a repetition and assimilation of the phase of separation (between nine months and three years). In these sorts of 'suns', there is not always a clear middle point but the direction of the rays point to the middle. The child often draws the rays interchangeably from outside to inside and from inside to outside.

We will later see that this form, the circle with rays, develops into a symbol of the sun in which the rays are drawn from the circle's edge and no longer through the edge. At about four, children begin to draw with more awareness. The sun with its rays first appears randomly all over the paper but, by the time the child is four, (if there is stabilization), the sun is given a fixed place at the top of the drawing on the left, in the middle or on the right. A face is almost always drawn in the sun. In this phase, this means that the child has become conscious of the natural world surrounding him. There is a feeling of certainty and warmth. More will be said about drawings of the sun in the chapter on the significance of the house.

Our ancestors did not know for certain if the sun would reappear each morning, just as the child in his or her first year of life does not know for certain if the mother will return after she has gone. Many myths tell of the daily setting of the sun that disappears into the underworld and is perhaps devoured but then returns in the morning. If the child is able to remember his or her mother and knows that she is somewhere else, separation can begin and the child can begin to safely explore the world. The way in which children draw a sun shows the extent to which the child has loosened the ties to the mother and the extent to which the protection by the external world, usually provided by the father, is present. For example, if a child older than six still draws a circle (or a sun) with rays that go through the edge of the circle or if the sun is still placed randomly on the paper, it may be that the child is still strongly tied to the mother. Such a child will not set out alone, shows little initiative and evidently still needs the protection of a mother(ly) figure. The separation as described in Mahler's theory has perhaps failed or has not been fully assimilated.

In the divine sun myths, the sun is independent of and free from the world. The sun is above everything and everyone; it sees everything and thus knows everything. The sun was the eye of God. In Jungian theory, the sun symbolizes the male process of becoming conscious and the separation from the mother. By male we mean the male function (the Animus), the force that is present in every man and woman that enables them to strive for expansion, action and connection.

The symbolism of the power and protection of the sun can be found in all cultures.

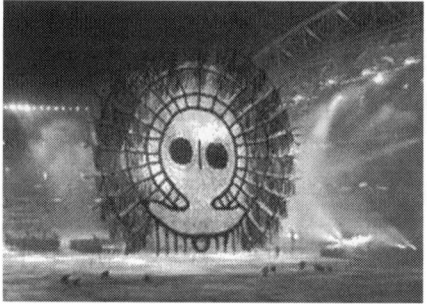

Opening of the Olympic Games 2002 Sydney

Being impressed by and afraid of natural phenomenon was part of the way of thinking common to our ancestors as they developed their consciousness. They experienced the cosmos and the overwhelming power of the natural world as divine powers. The gods were good or evil, they helped mankind or they punished them. For almost all primitive peoples, the sun represents a divine power.

4.10 Dots

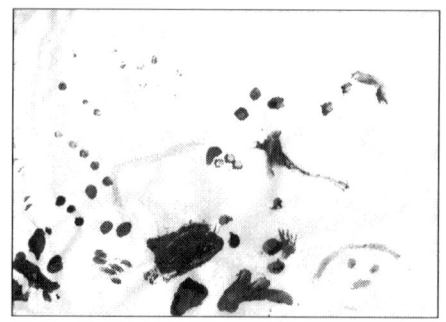 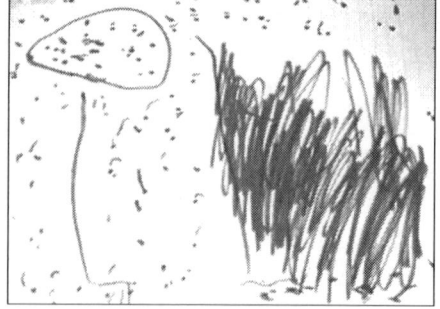

(girl, 3 years and 8 months)   *(boy, 4 years old)*

Description
Dots or points are spread across the paper. The dots are often part of a drawing.

Significance
The development of personal consciousness begins by becoming conscious of one's own body. The body is a source of life that will gradually acquire a spirit. The dots made with the fingertips are the fingerprints of the personality since the fingerprint contains unique

personal lines that can be used to identify an individual. Children of three or older can intentionally draw dots with a brush, a marker or their fingers.

A child becomes aware of rhythmic feelings in the course of the first year of life, and these are later expressed in a drawing as dots or points. These dots are often made by the child in a very lively and active manner, showing that the child is somewhat conscious of a certain liveliness inside himself, the biological clock, the rhythm of day and night, eating and sleeping. These are the predecessors of a sense of time and counting. We see that a child in this phase can feel the rhythm in music and dance and enjoys moving rhythmically, clapping his, nodding his head, etc. When making the dots, children often count and sing. This could be called the 'rhythm of time'. Chaos is followed by ordering, which is mythologically told in stories about the beginning of the world and the gods. From the beginning, 'Chaos', the time, 'Chronos', came into being.

Case illustration
The parents of a four-year-old girl asked my help in connection with sudden nightmares and stormy crying fits. Her father was often abroad for his work, sometimes for a few days and sometimes a few weeks. This had never been a problem, but the girl missed her father very much now. I advised the parents to make a sort of calendar with stickers and drawings to show the days when papa was at home and those when he was abroad. A few weeks after this had begun, the girl covered a sheet of paper with dots in different colours. She said to me, 'Now you have to count them.' She pointed to the dots according to colour and I had to count them. She showed that she had found a sort of rhythm and order in the chaos. The therapy could be terminated shortly thereafter.

Dots are a very old symbol. They were saved and became well-known by the Australian aboriginals. Modern man can no longer understand the meaning of these dots. Aboriginals call them drawings from the 'dream period', the period in which the spirits of the land and the ocean roamed over the earth bringing it life. (W. Kielich, *Volken en stammen*)

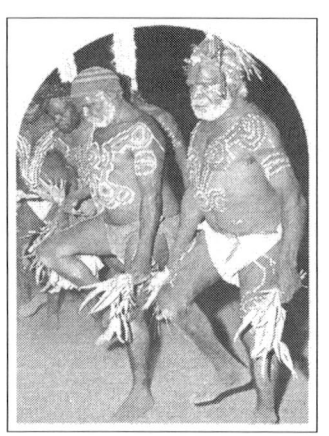 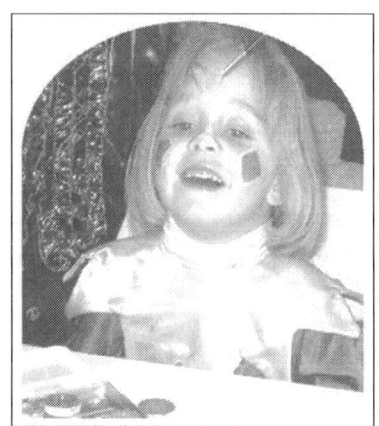

Tribal dances of Australian aboriginals with dots on their bodies

Carnival make-up

Drawings with dots point to the development of ego-consciousness. The child becomes increasingly conscious of himself or herself. This parallels the primitive phase of becoming conscious of the body that our ancestors experienced and expressed in decorating their bodies. The body drawings of the Australian aboriginals are still well known. The bodies of primitive peoples were decorated with tattoos in the form of group signs and were later individualized. Drawing on the body is a primitive stage leading to the use of a mask, which reinforced the wearer's personality. The personality was later further emphasized by clothes. And even today, our personalities are expressed in fashion, hairstyles and other external decorations.

When children draw on their bodies (hands, arms, legs), they give a sign of rediscovering and reinforcing the (bodily) personality. Make-up derives from this. Another unusual form of body decoration that we can see again today is drawing on the body by using tattoos. The deeper significance of such a body drawing is the attempt to come into contact via bodily feelings with a psychological ego-consciousness that stems from the phase in which our ancestors became conscious. It can be compared to the extensive manifestations in clothing and accessories that are used to reinforce one's personality. Although there is nothing wong with body painting as an art form, an exaggerated need to have sometimes painful tattoos (or piercing) or excessive body decorations can be an expression that covers an inner feeling of emptiness and an attempt to bring about an ego-consciousness.

4.11 Crosses

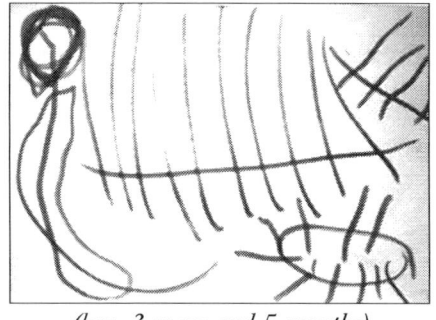

(boy, 3 years and 5 months)

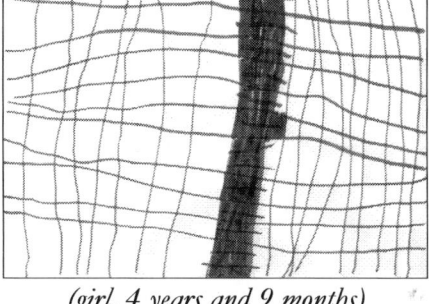

(girl, 4 years and 9 months)

Description
We can see lines crossing one another in the drawing.

Significance
Crossed lines point to the archetypal structure of spinning, weaving, knitting and plaiting, all typically activities for women. The crosses and the thread symbolize life and fate, and we speak of weaving a 'web of life' with the 'thread of life'.

Drawing lines that cross one another indicates a new phase. Crossed lines mean that choices can be made for a certain direction. The drawer makes lines on paper from left to right and from top to bottom. We also often see two long vertical lines with a number of small crosswise lines (a sort of ladder). The child has often literally experienced a cross period in which he or she intentionally crosses the opinions of others by saying 'no'. The child is becoming aware of his or her own purpose/goal. It is an important movement when a child has two lines cross each other. The child is then often more independent and psychologically stronger. There is a clear split in which the choice for a certain direction is made. An internal feeling of wanting to make choices fits in well with this period of saying 'no'. Rose Fleck says that a spinal column can be recognized in these sorts of crossed lines and that, in this period, the child's spinal column is stronger because he or she can walk independently; moreover, the child psychologically shows more 'backbone'.

In Egyptian hieroglyphics, the cross means 'new life' (*nem ankh*). Data analysis of this sign has shown that the cross is a combination of a sign for activity and a sign of passivity. Mythologically, the sign of the cross represents polarity and contradiction. There is also an important early significance of two crossing lines meaning fire and light since, in prehistoric times, man could make a fire by rubbing two sticks together. A cross is often drawn inside a circle (as a mandala) to show a growing ego consciousness.

In fairy tales, exploring and taking responsibilities for one's own deeds often begins as a person comes to a crossroads and must make a choice (e.g. Grimm's *Three Feathers*). The one who chooses the right direction in fairy tales is not always the cleverest but is rather often the character who is lazy or idle. The character usually allows himself to be led by his feeling and intuition, which later turns out to be the best choice. The fairy tale, as a source of human wisdom, tells us that, when making decisions, we should not always follow common sense but should listen to our inner feelings.

We look at how long and the extent to which a child draws these crosses. Are the lines drawn with confidence or with caution? Is the cross form in keeping with the child's age? In the case of some children, we may wonder if they find themselves in a period or circumstances in which they again have to make a choice. Or are they at the beginning of a new phase and desirous of going their own way?

We can see that children, especially adolescents who are in conflict with their parents, often draw complicated structures with connecting horizontal lines. By concentrating on the complicated structures and finding a way out, for example by demarcating the boundaries or 'crossing' lines, they can practice setting forth on their own path in a complicated real-life situation.

Case illustration

J. was a shy and quiet eleven-year-old boy with sudden temper tantrums that surprised others. The home situation was very complicated: an older sister was pregnant but continued to live at home, the parents argued a great deal and a younger brother was afraid to sleep by himself so J. and this brother had to go to bed at the same time. One day, J. wanted to play with a hammer; he found a piece of wood and some nails and drove large nails into the wood. Then he asked if I had thread. He wound a thin cotton thread around the heads of the nails and so formed a network of complicated design. In the middle of this net he placed a 'spider' made from a chestnut with wooden toothpicks. He hereby symbolically expressed that he had both the desire and the talent to make decisions about his own life. By picking up the 'thread' and weaving his own 'cloth', he was able to make his own 'clothes'. Following this, he was better able to express his wishes at home and to voice his opinions in conflict situations.

Young children who are in a difficult period or who experience complicated situations express conflicting inner feelings not only in their drawings but also in how they play; for example, they play with cars that collide with each other, they build roads that cross each other, they play with trains and cars that meet at rail crossings, planes take off and land from different runways, bridges are built so people and cars can go over and under them, swords are 'crossed' in duels. If we look closely at a child as he or she draws and plays, we can often understand them better. (*see also pg. 46*)

4.12   Balloons

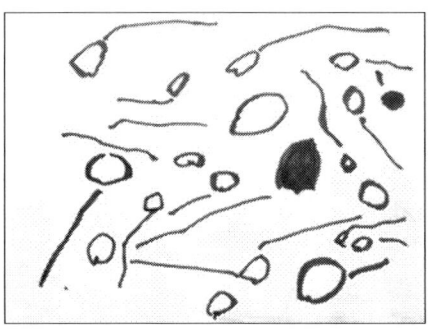

(*girl, 3 years and 2 months*)

Description
We can see circles and stripes that look like balloons (or sperm).

Significance

Toddlers and pre-school children often make drawings that look like balloons. These balloons can express the wish to become separate and to explore. Even at an early age, children are fascinated by balloons. If we describe a balloon as 'a thing that is held tightly and that nevertheless goes its own way', we can see how this expresses the inner experience of the child who is held by his or her mother – on a string so to speak – but who is free to explore the surrounding world.

The drawn balloon points to a phase of discovering the surroundings while still being somehow held by the mother, a phase common to the third and fourth years of life. The floating balloons can also be seen as expressions of wanting to make a choice for a certain direction, wanting to move off in every direction, wanting to find one's own way and wanting to be set loose. The first time that children experience this psychologically, they can stand straight and walk independently. They no longer stay within sight of the mother but go off on adventures. They actively explore their surroundings but still need support from someone familiar to them to whom they can return now and again. But they are learning to make themselves free, both physically and psychologically, of the ties that bind them to the mother. This is the age at which children experiment and go off on adventures and in which parents find themselves warning and watching cautiously. This phase is also expressed in games such as hide-and-seek or tag. Leaving and returning again are practised, experienced and expressed in a playful manner.

If we delve deeper, we could interpret this 'balloon feeling' as the first sense of liberation experienced by children immediately after birth. At birth, there is a desire to be freed (from the narrow passageway of the womb) and the relief felt when this succeeds (and the lungs are blown up with air so breathing can begin). If we see this together with the idea that the balloons also resemble sperm that, as we know, go off hunting in search of an egg cell, and considering that ejaculation is caused by desire and lust, we can also image that various layers of the psyche are combined in these balloon drawings.

In mythology, we find the wish to escape from being imprisoned, something that can be done only by flying, in the tale of Daedalus and his son Icarus. In his enthusiasm and carelessness, Icarus flew too close to the sun, causing the wax that held his wings together to melt so that, despite his father's warnings, he fell into the sea.

Floating and flying upwards point to the primordial wish to become separate from the father (and the mother). This myth tells us of youthful overconfidence that has to be channelled and halted because of the fatal consequences of going to high or too far. The child too must learn to find the middle path.

Case illustration
M. was a five-year-old girl who was put in the custody of another family when she was seven because her mother could not care for her. For quite some time, it was unclear whether or not she could remain with that family, partly because her mother has begun legal proceedings and partly because the children in the family found it difficult to accept her. It was eventually decided that M. could stay with the family. Good arrangements were made with the biological mother and the family situation became more peaceful. The girl filled a sheet of paper with balloons and drew a tree with a bird's nest in the same drawing. She evidently felt free and relieved as well as safe in a new nest!

If a child chooses a large number of balloons (and later also planes, birds, zeppelins, etc.) as the subject of his or her drawing, that can point to a desire to have more room or to be set free. The parents can try to decide if this wish can be granted. This same desire can sometimes be seen as an attempt to catch up if the feeling of becoming separate has not been fully assimilated. The balloon drawing can also be seen as a positive sign, an expression of relief and release after a period of having been stuck. We always have to view the drawing in the context of the child's phase of life and circumstances before we can say that there is a specific problem or conflict.

4.13 Coloured areas

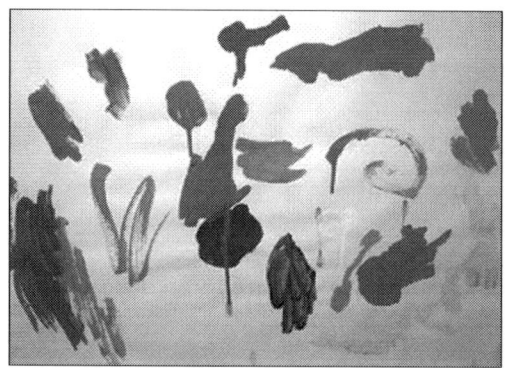

(girl, 4 years and 4 months.)

Description
We see various forms and colours spread across the entire sheet of paper.

Significance
If a child has successfully passed through the separation-individualization phase, he or she has achieved a certain stability. We can assume that a child of four has caught up with the past, and that the various phases of development have been assimilated in drawings and play. The child can now concentrate more on the present and the future, perhaps - and especially because - by assimilating and re-experiencing, the child has become surer of himself. Objects are given and retain a name. The child is aware of the immutability of things, that is, that object constancy has come into being: the child knows that the mother is there even when she is physically absent. The child can retain the presence of the mother in his thoughts and has thus no problems with this.

Working towards this phase, the child uses the paper more consciously, draws more consciously, colours with pleasure and enjoys finishing a drawing. We can see in the child's behaviour and play that he she enjoys using a space and making new discoveries. This can be compared to the balanced, spacious and colourful drawings of children at the age of about four. The child feels comfortable with the space on the paper and places a colour or a form wherever he or she wants to. The child has drawn all of the basic forms and is able, in principle, to draw whatever he or she wishes.

In these drawings with filled areas, we can see how a child feels in relation to his or her surroundings. For example, if we see that a child fills in only a very small corner of the paper, it could mean that the child is uncertain about whether or not he or she may be somewhere else. If we see that a child of four still repeatedly draws beyond the edges of the paper, it means that the child still experiences a certain boundlessness. This can be an inner boundlessness caused by insufficient psychological growth, but also the result of an unstructured living situation caused by the external world. The use of just one or a few colours despite having every colour available can point to a certain one-sidedness or lack of vitality. This will be discussed in more depth in the chapter about the symbolic significance of colours.

4.14   Smearing and messing about

(boy, 4 years and 2 months)

Description
Finger paint drawing in which all of the colours are mixed together, resulting in brown or grey.

Significance
From about the age of two onwards, children are increasingly interested in defecating and urinating. At about the age of three, most children are potty-trained so that they can use a potty or the toilet. This phase also has its physical and a psychological significance. Children must be capable of keeping something of themselves inside, excreting it and then taking a distance from it. The problems in this phase are often connected to a power struggle, stubbornness and not being able to let go of underlying feelings.

This is the emotional world that gives rise to messy games such as playing with mud or clay, finger painting, playing with food, etc. These sorts of games show the child that something changes by moving and mixing, and children experience a sense of power because these changes are caused by their own hands. On the one hand, there is a change in material and colour brought about by the child himself and, on the other hand, the child has to experience and accept the fact that changes can happen spontaneously. This process can be compared to the feeling of control that has to be given up when a child defecates. Because the faeces leaves the body from the back, the child cannot see it, making it even more frightening since it seems to happen spontaneously. Children are usually not allowed to play with their faeces because it is dirty, and rightly so! Playing with mud, clay or finger paints approaches the feeling of touching and playing with faeces. Most children between the ages of three and five enjoy using finger paints.

If children repeatedly make dirty painting over a longer period of time, play preferably with soft clay, or sit constantly in the mud, this can mean that certain conflicts that arose during potty-training still have to be resolved. As a parent or care provider, we can try to discover which problems these could have been and try to find a solution (for example, by taking a different attitude in a particular conflict).

Case illustration
B. was a seven year old boy who came for therapy because he had eating problems. Since the age of three (around the time of potty-training) he had refused to eat a warm meal. He nibbled on cheese and crackers and ate a lot of sweets. Family dinners were a disaster: there were always arguments because the boy said that everything was 'dirty'. I was not surprised when he often chose finger paints so he could mix all of the colours together. He made some 'deliciously dirty dinners' from some of my soft yellow clay. It looked like faeces. He called his dish 'dirty spinach'. He had me pretend to taste it and ate some of it himself. 'Dirty, isn't it?' We laughed a lot about this. Shortly after this, his mother told me that he had begun to eat warm meals again. His conflict between eating and defecating had been symbolically expressed and could be assimilated in a playful fashion.

4.15 Colouring in pages of a colouring book

From the age of about three or four, children enjoy colouring in a colouring book. Some parents worry that this will not sufficiently stimulate the child's fantasy. They do not approve of the activity because they do not find it creative. But colouring in a colouring book has a special and valuable significance. The child must physically be capable of holding a pencil and colouring in a certain direction so that he or she does not go past the lines of the figure. Intellectually, the child must be able to recognize the figures both as a whole (what is this drawing about?) and in detail (what is included and what colours are associated with these details?). From the viewpoint of behavioural psychology, the child must be able to keep himself within the drawn lines. The child must also be able to picture reality. He wants to and is able to follow the rules; he knows how it should be. The standards of the schoolroom and the family become more important for children. This need for order is often present from about the sixth year when children want to know how things should be or must be. Colouring books are also popular if the drawings are of subjects that the child is currently interested in, such as Disney figures or fantasy figures with which the child plays. Drawings that are connected to holidays (Christmas, Easter, etc.) also fit into the child's world. We can examine if and how a child colours in these drawings from a physical, intellectual or psychological point of view. We can also see the extent to which the child is adjusted and if he or she is able to and wants to follow the rules of the game. This is something that most children who are able to go to kindergarten or pre-school can do from the age of four.

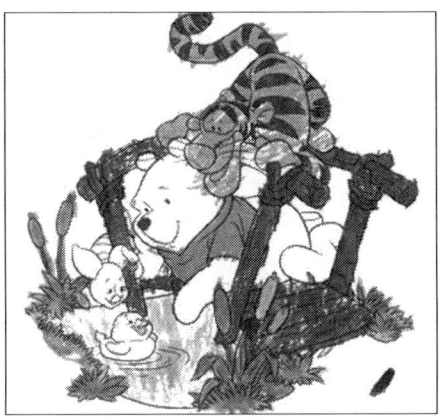

It is also possible that, in periods of uncertainty, children prefer to colour in drawings that have already been made. A ready-made drawing offers safety, structure and boundaries, and it is clear what the drawing is about. Colouring within the lines demands a certain amount of control, and having control over the hands and the body means that the child has some control over a situation. Spontaneous drawings demand too much energy if feelings are blocked. It is sometimes necessary that a child finds a way to repair his internal control. He keeps to his own natural boundaries which parents should recognize and respect. But children can sometimes be stimulated to make a spontaneous drawing if they colour ready-made drawings too frequently or if they colour nothing else except these. The child may tend to stick to the same fixed patterns. We can see the extent to which a child who draws like this is giving us a sign.

Case illustration

P. was nine years old when she came down with a serious illness that hospitalized her for several weeks. She was finally allowed home, where she followed a strict diet and took a great amount of medicine. For weeks after this, she only coloured in colouring books or drew the same Donald Duck figure. She could draw spontaneously only after she had returned to school and was used to her new lifestyle.

CHAPTER 5

CHILDREN DRAW THEMSELVES

5.1 The significance of the tadpole

In this chapter we will discuss the significance of drawings of human figures made by children between the ages of two to about seven. These figures show that the awareness of the body is in keeping with awareness of the psyche. Man was capable of developing a self-awareness by becoming aware of his own body; he attached significance to various sensations in the body. The child goes through this same process in the first few years of childhood. By looking at a drawing of a human figure made by a child, who spontaneously depicts himself or herself in the drawing, we can often see how the child feels and if there are physical or psychological problems or conflicts.

C.G. Jung and E. Neumann were the first to make a link between the evolutionary development of the human psyche and the psychological development of the child. Nowadays, there are evolution psychologists who discover and describe relations with the (especially biological) history of mankind and the present behaviour of humans (Steven Pinkers, Robert Wrights). Various psychological theories have come increasingly closer together now that earlier hypothetical assumptions about the human psyche have been confirmed by physics, biology and mathematics.

The descriptions of the significance of children's drawings given in this chapter take into consideration the relationship between the body and the psyche. In addition, we will also look at similarities between these drawings and mythological stories and how they relate to evolutionary theories and modern theories of behavioural and developmental psychology.

The evolution of the tadpole into a complete human is drawn by children from various cultures in the same way (Kellogg). Most adults recognize the tadpole: a drawing of a circle with short lines. Tadpoles begin after the phase of drawings spirals and simultaneously with the first attempts to draw a circle. When describing this figure, the child often says, 'That's me' or 'It's a little child'. When describing the evolution of the drawings of human figures, we must be aware of the fact that, as with the forms described in the previous chapter, these figures are not always drawn according to a fixed pattern. Although a toddler usually begins to draw a tadpole at about the age of two, they can be drawn for a long time after this as well.

We can follow the physical and psychological functions of the child in the development of details in the figures. The child knows that he or she has various bodily parts with various functions. During the first years of childhood, children discover their physical feelings, and these bodily feelings induce the development of the psyche, as also occurred with their ancestors before them. These discoveries can be seen in the first drawings of human figures. Children also know what is allowed and what is not, and the conscience can now develop. These drawings are universal because they reflect the normal, healthy basic development of the child.

Some of the intelligence tests still in use, such as Draw-A-Person, assess the 'logical level of development rather than the child's personality' (Otto Gmelin). In this test for children, the number of details in a drawing of a person is counted. Although it is generally true that the more details the further the intelligence has developed, the number of details can be influenced by emotional factors. Special signals, such as an emphasis on or absence of certain details or an incomplete human figure, can provide us with information about the child's psychological and physical condition. Although such signals are, however, random impressions, parents or others who recognizes them should be made aware of possible problems, conflicts or disturbances. A signal can be compared to a symptom, such as a headache. It may be insignificant, the child might be tired or feel unwell, but if such signals appear often, we should pay attention and try to discover the cause.

It is completely normal that a child one day draws complete figures standing next to a house and a tree and that, on the following day, he or she draws only circles or crosses. And on yet another occasion, the child may just scribble all over the paper or revert to drawing spirals or some of the other forms previously discussed. This may mean that these forms and the significance related to them must be repeated in the child's daily life. It is both logical and natural that these earliest basic forms and the basic feelings associated with them have to be repeated again and again to anchor them securely in the child's emotional life.

Because it is possible to follow and recognize the psychological and physical development of a child in these drawings of people, it is interesting to examine the drawings closely and to understand the meaning of each detail. If we do this well, we will recognize the behaviour and the significance of the drawings in the normal daily life of the child. We can see that the child has learned something new or has become stuck in a certain pattern of behaviour. Sometimes, drawings announce the imminent beginning of a certain development. But we cannot expect these drawings to act as a fortune teller's magic ball. It demands insight and experience to recognize normal, healthy developments in children's drawings and to understand their significance. Only then can we recognize special signals or abnormalities.

5.2   Tadpole

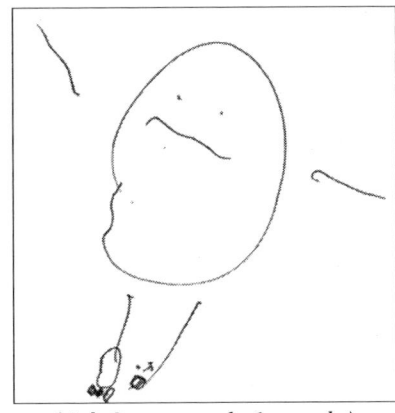 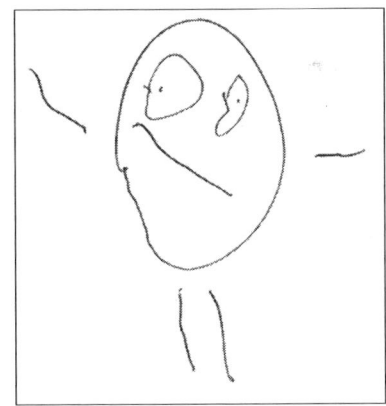

(girl, 2 years and 6 months)   *(boy, 2 years and 9 months)*

Description
A circle containing little circles for the eyes and a stripe for the mouth. Unconnected to the head, lines for arms and/or legs.

71

Significance
The head and the body are still experienced as one whole. At the beginning, a child draws a head in remembrance of the time that he or she could not yet distinguish between head and body. As we know, the first contacts with the external world are experienced by the head. Looking, tasting, hearing and smelling are the senses found in the head, and the mouth is the most important organ of contact. Not just food, but everything is explored with the mouth in the first few months of life, the period that Freud calls the 'oral phase'. We can also call this the 'pre-verbal' phase because things, people and feelings do not yet have names. The child tastes, hears, feels and smells, but does not recognize these functions as his or her own. In the first few months after birth, the person who cares for the child is a sort of container of these functions; the child gradually makes these functions his own as he begins to differentiate between himself and the other.

This experience is similar to the psychological prehistory of mankind. Early man began to think about himself only after he became conscious of his own body and his surroundings. Because breathing, eating, seeing and hearing happened with the head, the head was considered to be the basis of life. For a long time, the head remained the most important part of the psyche. Thoughts and feelings entered the head via the breath. Words, as expressions of these thoughts, also left the head via the breath. Feelings were also transported by the breath from inside to outside and back again. The word 'emotion' derives from the word *emovere*, meaning 'moving from inside to outside'. In Greek, the word 'psyche' means 'breath, air' (O.R. Broxton). Even today, we can still see that emotions are expressed via the head and the mouth. It is universal body language to grasp one's head in an intensely emotional moment or to clap one's hands over one's mouth as if the emotions might otherwise be spit out.

From earliest times, mankind thought that the psyche was located in the head; today, we know that the psyche is not just in the mind but throughout the body. The physical and psychological development of the child shows us that there is no distinction between psyche and body, but that this is an indivisible relationship. The distinction that people still sometimes want to make between body and psyche contradicts the experience that psychological reactions may occur in all parts of the body. Our stomachs turn if we are afraid or tense, and our legs turn to jelly if we find ourselves caught in a traumatic situation.

Physical and psychological aspects have always played a role in the child's relationship with his or her mother. Not only bodily care but also love, attention and the feeling of being welcome are existential values for a child, a precondition to surviving. That it is difficult to imagine the psyche is a typically human trait arising from the fact that we cannot fully comprehend the contents and function of the psyche. Philosophers, religions, scientists, physicists, psychiatrists and psychologists have all studied this issue. We cannot examine the various viewpoints and theories about the meaning of the psyche here. Some people deny the existence of a psyche, whereas others say they are fully familiar with it. What we can do is to describe the psychological functions of these drawings as clearly as possible, without being restrictive or subjective and using analytical studies and insights such as those discussed in the previous chapters.

5.3 Tadpole with a belly

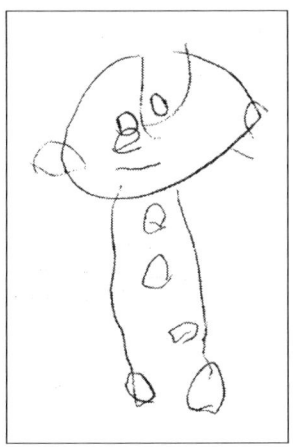

(girl, 2 years and 3 months)

Description
We see a head with eyes, nose, mouth and ears. There are two vertical lines with little feet and, between them, one or more circles.

Significance
The drawing of the tadpole with arbitrarily placed limbs is followed by the tadpole with legs extending vertically downwards. This expresses the

experience of the baby who suddenly finds arms and legs appearing in his or her range of vision. We can also see that something exists between the legs, the beginnings of an abdomen. The head has a number of details, but the rest of the body just dangles beneath it. The first things drawn after the head are the arms and legs, which is logical since these limbs are always moving and quickly come into the child's range of vision. The baby also becomes aware that part of his or her body, the stomach, can be the source of various sensations such as hunger, satisfaction or pain.

In chapter five of his book *The Child, the family and the outside world*, the English child psychologist D.W. Winnicot describes the baby's relation with his or her abdomen and small stomach, a part of the body that plays an important role in whether or not the baby feels content. The air in a full stomach has to be released by burping. Mothers pat their babies on the back to produce these little bubbles of air. Do the dots or circles between the legs perhaps represent these little burps? The child feels that the stomach is somewhere between the head and the legs; he or she is also aware that something enters the stomach and that something leaves. In this drawing, we see that the rump of the body is open. The underside of the stomach is evidently not yet felt since the child cannot consciously hold on to what is in the stomach. The body is still open, and the child is not yet potty-trained.

5.4   Head and rump

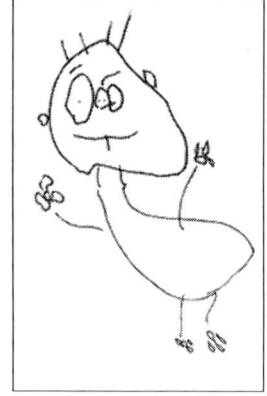 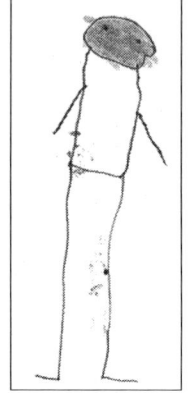

(girl, 4 years and 3 months.)   *(boy, 4 years and 5 months.)*

Description
More details are drawn. We can see a head, body, legs, arms, hands and feet.

Significance

The distinction now made between head, body and legs is the following step in the development of the child's physical awareness. A child who is aware of his or her own body often has more self-confidence, and children who are self-confident are often more intelligent. We also see that girls draw their bodies as a round shape, whereas boys draw a square body. This is because, at this age, boys and girls have become aware of physical differences. We can again see this difference between boys and girls between three and four in the games they play. Whereas boys play with building blocks and often make a tower, girls who play with the blocks often build round structures. Freudian psychologists say that boys are expressing their phallic fantasies and girls their vaginal functions. But we also recognize the primordial artistic custom, common to all cultures, of expressing the woman as round (a vase) and the man as tall and square (totem). The most primitive expression of the human body was that of a vat in which food could be stored. When man became aware of the sexual differences between men and women, this vat became the special symbol of the female, who could store new life in her body. The strength and vitality of the male was expressed in a tall, square form. We will return to this in detail when discussing how children draw genitals.

If a closed rump is drawn it usually means that the child has become potty-trained and that the contents of the body can be kept inside. Being able to retain and release faeces and urine coincides with the ability to control psychological impulses and to cope with tension. Normal potty-training takes this into account. The need to have control over a situation fits into the conflict between giving and taking, releasing and retaining. If potty-training takes too long or has to be repeated, it could point to circumstances that a child cannot control. A new baby, moving house or other such changes may result in tension that causes the child to wet his or her pants again.

It is possible that intelligent children draw human figures with fewer details if, for example, they have been ill or have had an accident that causes the child to experience his or her own body as traumatic. In addition, an inner feeling of uncertainty may also be expressed.

Case illustration

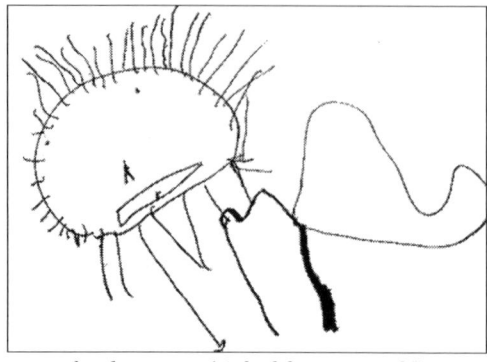
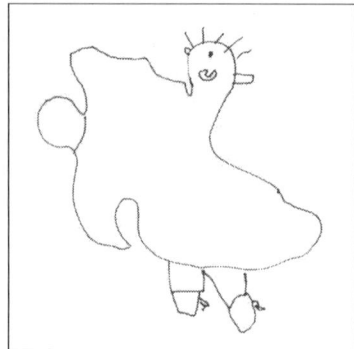

broken arm (girl of five years old)   *insecure (girl of four years old)*

A five-year-old girl fell off her scooter and broke her arm, which was then set in a plaster cast. In the drawing she shows how she feels.

A four-year-old girl had just heard that she was going on holiday together with her father. Although she was happy, she was also uncertain because she would not see her mother for a while. Although she could previously draw figures very well, in this drawing she appears disorganized and shows her uncertainty.

5.5 The pre-school child and magical thinking

As toddlers and pre-schoolers, children prefer to play alone or with two or three other children. As they discover the world around them, they imitate it: playing house, store, doctor, etc. They also use animals, real or stuffed toys, in their games. This is the period of the most important phase of magical thinking (Selma Fraiburg). The child has a rich imagination in which animals and events can take on magical qualities. This is logical if you realize that the child knows only a small part of reality and that, unhindered by any further knowledge, creates his or her own reality. This may cause the most natural things to become sources of fear (the sound of the wind, shadows on the wallpaper, etc.). Pre-schoolers begin to learn what they may and may not do and begin to form standards and values as well as a conscience. All the rules set down by their parents and others may cause feelings of guilt, which, in turn, lead to fear. The child may think that his or her thoughts can be heard by someone else. Fear is a normal phenomenon in children; fear is needed so that children can express themselves and control their fear. Fear diminishes as consciousness and the intellect grow. Intellectually, the child begins to learn a great deal about reality by asking questions (the so-called 'why' phase).

It is a known fact that our ancestors attributed magical qualities to the world around them. Spirits were found in trees and there were holy places with miraculous powers. They also attributed these magical qualities to animals and other people. What we today call a game of fantasy was serious business for our ancestors. The primitive dancers who used masks were playing as if they were the animal in the mask. People believed, for example, that the spirit of a deceased person was in that animal, giving rise to a certain feeling of communion with the animal's spirit. In this way, man came into touch with animal instincts and, unconsciously, with his own natural instincts. This was necessary in order to learn what his own feelings were.

We call such actions 'projections' because the personal inner content is projected onto objects and people in the external world. Such magical thinking can still be found today in, for example, the symbolism of the national flag, a soccer club or a pop idol. No one may disfigure or insult these symbols because people or groups identify with them. In general, people are aware of the significance of these feelings. The transition from belief in magic to acknowledging the facts could take place only when man had become conscious of his surroundings and after he had developed his ability to think. The magical phase is a forerunner of personal consciousness. Intellectual growth enables man to look more objectively at himself.

Being able to draw a human figure is a good sign of the development of individuality; by drawing themselves, children are able to project themselves onto the external world. Children who draw themselves become increasingly aware of themselves and, as this awareness grows, the drawings of human figures contain increasingly more details. This process is similar to primitive man's gradually becoming more aware of his body and assigning it a psychological significance.

The child's growing awareness of his body and bodily functions is similar to the growth of the development of his psyche. We can see the growth of both physical and psychological awareness in the details of drawings of human figures discussed below. We should try to image that, as our ancestors gradually became conscious of their bodies, they were able to use this awareness to explain psychological manifestations. The indivisible connection between body and psyche that our ancestors experienced as a given truth also applies to the developing child. It is not true that modern adults have lost this connection, but rather that they do not experience it as such.

5.6 Details in drawings of human figures

- **The mouth**

The mouth is first drawn as a line, but details such as lips and teeth are soon included so that the mouth can express a positive or a negative emotion (a laughing or crying mouth).

Significance

The mouth, one of the most important parts of the head, is central to breathing, eating, speaking and expression. Facial expression is known in the apes (Center for Nonverbal Studies, Washington) and has long been evolutionarily anchored in humans.

Eating is essential to being able to exist and survive. It is the first need that humans express and need to satisfy. The baby uses his or her mouth to discover food, the mother, the breast or the nipple of a bottle. He or she uses the mouth to explore all sorts of objects and materials. Throughout life, loving contact occurs via the mouth, the lips being the most sensitive organ of intimate contact.

Teeth enable us to devour tougher food, which may explain the aggressive significance of teeth in the mouth. As explained in the earlier discussion of the tadpole, the mouth is very important in expressing feelings (air, breath, psyche), which is why children pay special attention to drawing the mouth. With the mouth they can express their experiences of eating, talking, love, fear, aggression, sadness, surprise, etc.

- **Hair**

Hair is usually drawn as little lines on top of the head. As children become aware of their own sex, girls are drawn with long hair and boys with short.

Significance

Hair has always signified strength because hair grows quickly, is very strong and does not decay. In the beginning, the hair that is drawn corresponds to the development the ego. Hair that is emphatically drawn points to a strong cognitive function; there are a great many things going on in that head, perhaps too many in some children! By drawing lines on top of the head, children show that they consciously or unconsciously experience the fact that there is an activity somewhere up in the head. Hair grows day and night, just as do thoughts that arise during the day and at night in our dreams. Hair often plays an important role in fairy tales, mythology and religion (the colour, whether or not it is cut off, etc.).

In children's drawings, girls are usually drawn with long hair and boys with short. Although the styles may vary, children usually follow this rule. From about the age of seven, children begin to draw themselves and others more realistically and they are then more aware of their own hairstyles as part of their personalities, as is also true of decorations and clothes on the body. Children from countries around the Mediterranean Sea often draw women with a veil and men with a moustache or a beard. The veil covers the hair, which has long been a symbol of sexuality. In Egypt, a long braid was a sign of youth and long hair a sign of virginity, whereas facial hair was a sign of a man's (sexual) strength and wisdom.

- **Eyes**

If we see two little circles next to each other in a larger circle, then we assume that this is a drawing of a face, especially if there is a small line underneath the circles that seems to be a mouth.

Significans

The eyes and the mouth are the most important facial features. The intense eye contact between a mother and her child in the first hours after birth is important in establishing a good relationship. Research has shown that babies look into their mothers' eyes even when the mother is speaking.

From about the age of four, children draw an extra dot or little circle in the eye: the pupil. Eyes without pupils have a blank expression; the pupil gives the eye a soul. The word 'pupil' originally meant 'young child'. If you look closely at the pupil, you will see a very small person. Our ancestors thought that everyone carried a small person within them, which is why they called this part of the eye the pupil. If children draw a pupil, this indicates a growing self-awareness. Empty eyes make it difficult to establish contact. In drawings of humans done by older children (from about the age of seven), empty eyes may indicate a sense of inner emptiness, but they may also indicate developmental disorders problems in making contact such as happens, for example, with forms of autism. Children usually draw eyes that are looking straight ahead, but they sometimes draw eyes looking to the left or to the right. Looking aside like this may indicate shyness or insecurity, but we should not draw conclusions about this without first examining the child's actual situation.

- **Nose**

In the tadpole, the nose is drawn at almost the same time as the eyes and the mouth. As a child develops, he or she discovers many ways of trying to draw a three-dimensional nose: small lines, squares, triangles, nostrils, etc.

Significance

Drawing the nose is not a problem, but what is unusual is if a child does not draw a nose. We then have to ask ourselves why the nose is missing. The nose is the most primitive organ used to orient ourselves in the world. Our animal ancestors used their noses to find food and meet a partner. A newborn baby recognizes his mother's smell and, when put on the mother's stomach, the baby turns towards the breasts for milk. A smell can bring back a long-forgotten moment. Consciously and unconsciously, smells always play a role in contact between human beings. This is why it is so noticeable if a child does not add a nose to his or her drawing of a human being or if the nose is strangely drawn. There may be a relation between this and a possible disturbance in the primary contact between mother and child, but negative physical experiences (a nose operation, a bloody nose) or being mistreated (pinched by the nose) may also reasons for the nose being 'forgotten' or unusual.

- **Neck**

From about the age of six, children begin to draw the neck separately as vertical lines between the head and the rump.

Significance

The distinction between head (the intellect) and body (feelings) is underlined. The will has developed, and the neck enables the child to turn his or her head in all directions.

If the neck is emphasized, it may mean that internal and bodily impulses are being held under control and that the child is acting primarily via the intellect (the head). In non-verbal communication, supporting the neck with the hands is a sign of uncertainty that has evolved from the gesture used to protect the most vulnerable part of the body, the neck, from attack by another animal of prey. If after the age of seven a child does not draw a neck, it may mean that the person has no control over his or her own will (little willpower) or that the child's will is being suppressed by, for example, a strong authority.

- **Ears**

The ears may be drawn at an early age.

Significance

As openings in the head, ears are organs that enable an exchange between the internal and the external world. The ears hear what may and may not be said. A child's conscience can now be formed. Ears are drawn when the child begins to consciously listen. If a child forgets to draw ears, it may indicate that he or she does not want to hear something. And large ears may mean that the child enjoys listening to, for example, what adults say to one another.

- **Hands**

Hands can be drawn in various sizes and with fingers.

Significance

Hands connect us to the outside world; we come into contact with people and material by touching and feeling. In many cultures, the first conscious social contact with other individuals is made with the hands. At an early age, children learn to wave with their hands or to shake hands. The attention given to the hand in a drawing reflects the way in which the child is in contact with other people. Proportionally large hands may indicate aggression from and towards the external world. Hands that are too small or that are hidden behind the back, for example, or in pockets may indicate shyness or problems in social contacts. Fingernails that are emphatically drawn may indicate aggressive emotions since, in the course of evolution, nails have been the aggressive animal element with which an animal holds its prey.

- **Fingers and toes**

The child becomes increasingly aware of the complete body, especially if the child counts the five fingers and toes while drawing them.

Significance

The number five is an old and meaningful symbol. It is the number of the complete physical, material, natural human being consisting of a rump and four limbs. The brains are now aware of a new physical status, which is why new mental changes can occur. For example, children can now speak well and understandably and they can count to five. If a child makes a mistake in the number of fingers or toes that he or she draws, it may be that something is bringing the child out of balance.

- **Feet**

Feet are first drawn as stripes and round toes. Shoes are drawn later.

Significance

We are connected to the earth when we stand and walk. We can use our feet to move freely and independently. The foot as a footprint means that something has been occupied as property. When children begin to walk upright, their view of the world expands. Walking upright is the first evolutionary difference between humans and animals. From the time that man began to walk upright, he began to develop intellectually. We are familiar with the old expression of being treated 'like a doormat', a sign of being submissive. Placing a foot on a prisoner of war, slaves or disobedient servants was a sign of how much they were held in despise.

In children's drawings, the foot shows us how children stand in relation to the world around them. This can be with small, thin feet or with large, strong feet. A foot that can be used to kick (aggression) or 'not having a leg to stand on'. No feet or standing on only one leg may be a sign of dependence or imbalance. The shoes on the feet can also add to the significance of the feet. Large, strong shoes with sharp points or heels or invisible shoes that give very little support. Shoes can be a weapon or they can help to express or strengthen a personality. All of this shows us how a child stands in relation to the world.

- **Knees**

Children often draw knees with special emphasis, which is unusual because this rarely occurs with other joints such as elbows, wrists, etc.

Significance

The word 'knee' derives from the Latin *genu*, which means 'source'. According to *The Origins of European Thought* by Richard Onians, the knees were the seat of strength and vitality. This can be attributed to man's realizing that he was strong and vital for as long as he could move his knees. A second meaning of the knee being a 'source' could perhaps derive from the fact that, in earlier times, women gave birth while kneeling, which may have promoted the knee being referred to as the 'source'. In many cultures and religions, kneeling is a gesture of respect for one's superior; even today, it is customary to kneel before religious and royal leaders. This psychological explanation helps us to understand that children in a certain phase of life draw knees with emphasis. If a child draws firmly locked knees it may mean that he or she does not want to be brought to their knees by a person or an idea.

- **Navel**

A dot or a little circle drawn exactly in the middle of the abdomen. Later, the dots or circles are drawn one underneath the other, and the child calls them 'buttons'. Usually not more than eight buttons are drawn.

Significance

The navel is usually located in the middle of the body. It is through the navel that the unborn child receives oxygen and food. The umbilical cord binds the child to the mother, a tie that is abruptly severed at birth but that remains visible in the navel. Psychologically, the toddler and the pre-school child see their own ego, connected with the mother, as the centre of the world. In mythology, we find the 'navel of the world' as a symbol for the centre of the world. There is the famous stone in the Temple at Delphi that was considered the 'navel of the earth', and more navel stones have been found, ranging from the Islamic Kaaba to the navel stones in Jerusalem. Depictions of the navel have therefore an archetypal significance, a universal human significance that has arisen from a universal natural experience.

If a child of pre-school age or older draws a navel, it may mean that the child still has strong emotional ties to the mother. At about the age of six, the navel as a symbol of egocentricity is replaced by a number of buttons that are drawn in a straight line from top to bottom. The number of buttons often coincides with the child's age. It is not completely clear why almost all children draw these buttons and why they stop doing so after about the age of eight. Perhaps they then realize that other people also have an Ego. Many adults can remember the moment in their childhood when they became aware of the fact that other people had an Ego just as they did (Kohnstam). The row of buttons in the drawing could mean that the child is still convinced of his or her own uniqueness. When this egocentric manner of thinking is abandoned, the new personality can be expressed in clothes and detailed fashion.

- **Clothing**

Children usually begin to draw clothes at about the age of six. Sometimes, they draw details of an article of clothing on the abdomen (decorations on a sweater or a belt).

Significance

From the moment that the child is aware of and accepts his or her own sex, a boy or a girl is drawn wearing clothes. Because in today's fashion both boys and girls wear long pants, children draw the same clothes for both sexes. But since girls usually wear brighter colours and since they also wear a dress now and again, there are also drawings with coloured and decorated dresses. Clothes give a certain status and show other people who you are. Detailed clothing that includes sleeves, collars and edging indicates a strong personality. The child is aware of himself and can underline this in his clothing. Drawing detailed clothing also expresses a sense of being part of a community (the collective). Children see and know what sort of clothing is worn by other children and they want to participate and belong to this community in which they can also express their own preferences.

- **Headgear**

From about the age of six, both boys and girls draw men with a hat and women with long hair.

Significance

A hat or a cap emphasizes the personality. The child is more aware of his or her own identity. Hats have always been a sign of power, both among the original inhabitants of America, where the Indian chief wore the largest feathers, and among royalty with their crowns. The most important person makes himself taller by wearing something on his head. The hat that was higher than someone else's hat was a symbol of a higher status and personal power.

Today, both boys and girls of a certain age enjoy wearing a baseball cap. The cap is a sign of wanting to feel stronger and of trying to hide any insecurity by wearing something 'cool'. In the Western world, women still wear hats on special occasions to emphasize their personalities (as mother of the bride, at a royal reception, at horse races and in official political functions). Men rarely wear hats, not even on official occasions; they do wear a hat or cap if it is functional, for example, as protection against the sun or the cold. And there is the cap that is worn as a sort of uniform outfit at demonstrations as a sign of solidarity. In the early years of women's emancipation (late 19th and early 20th centuries), women's hats were adorned with exceptionally large feathers. Status and power were relatively new for women, which may explain why hats for women are still more common than are hats for men. Are women perhaps (unconsciously) trying to catch up?

Nevertheless, children still draw sex-specific headgear and hairstyles (see also the significance of *hair*) as a sign that they are not yet as emancipated as are their own parents. But this comes in puberty.

- **Genitals**

From about the age of five or six, children openly begin to draw sexual signals. Girls draw breasts and a vagina, boys draw a phallus. This is true not only when they draw themselves but also when they draw their parents (or brother or sister).

Significance

Drawing sexual traits points to a recognition and acceptance of one's own sexual identity.

Primitive people often depict the genitals in their statues or drawings. A pregnant abdomen, breasts and the phallus represent bodily traits that distinguish a man from a woman. New life came from the vagina. But it is generally assumed that early man was not aware that sexual pleasure and intercourse were connected to the child that grew in the woman's abdomen. This is similar to young children who, although they experience sexual feelings, do not connect them to sexual relations or pregnancy.

Primitive man did notice the difference between male and female characteristics in nature when he began to work the soil. Nature was an example of human, natural and physical traits. The earth was the example of the female body; it was a dark cavity where seeds came to life and it provided nourishment for this life. The fertility of the earth was probably used as an example to understand the fertility of a woman. People saw that water was needed to make the earth fertile. Women searched for plants, sowed seeds and harvested the plants and herbs. They made vats from clay to store their oil and wine under the ground. The men were examples of activity and strength during the hunt. They did the heavy work and built the huts and the boats. They made contact with strangers and enemies in distant places. Nature was again the example used to understand the male nature. The phallus became a sign of strength and growth. As man developed intellectually, he was able to make connections between intercourse and offspring. The matriarchal period in which female (fertility) gods were revered because they were thought to have knowledge of life and death was followed by the patriarchal period. Under the influence of religions and male domination, the strength of women was suppressed and denied. The female body was considered to be a barren field that could become productive only after the male had sown his seed. It was not until the last century that women massively and openly demonstrated and demanded to be recognized as full individuals next to and equal to men. The psychological realization of the equality of women is parallel to the realization and biological knowledge of the natural physical characteristics of the human body with regard to sexuality and reproduction.

Drawing genitals at the age of six or seven fits into the awakening sex-specific consciousness of the child and has no sexual significance. After the age of nine, drawn sexual symbols are a sign demanding further attention, especially if the child has already been told a bit about sex.

5.7 Learning to look at a drawing of a human being

It is clear that each drawing by each child is unique. The purpose of the examples given below is to demonstrate how to look at the details in the drawing of a human being and to find both their general and their personal significance. Looking closely will give us insight.

The conclusions in the practical examples discussed below have not been drawn too precisely because that would involve disclosing too many private facts, which is not necessary in the framework of this study. Even without having exact information about the background of the drawer, an examination of the details in a drawing will still give us indications of the structure of the drawer's personality.

Case illustration 1

A drawing by a seven-year-old boy, the youngest in a family of three boys.

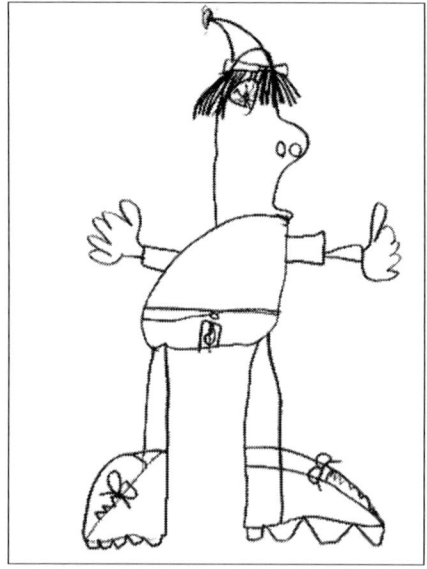

drawing of a person (seven-year-old boy)

Let us examine this drawing from the top to the bottom.

The *first impression* is that there is a pointed hat on the head. It is a hat that does not befit a boy of seven. Perhaps the imagination is (too) childish (an elf's hat) or the figure is a joker (a clown), but it could also be a nightcap. Or perhaps the child is emphasizing the head because so much happens there. The stripes of the hair also point to a lot of activity in the head. That could signify intelligence but also a great imagination. The head could also have been drawn in profile by using a skill learned from classmates or older children, which is normal for this age (the group standard).

The *face* does not look at us frontally. The person looks to the right, which usually means that he will orient himself to reality and will choose his own path. But this is true only of the head and not (yet) of the rest of the body, which could mean that the person wants to do something but he cannot (yet). The *mouth* is wide open, which could indicate an emphatic oral need (like eating sweets) or talking a lot (screaming) to express emotions. The *ears* have not been drawn, which could mean that he does not listen well or that he does not want to hear certain things.

We see that there is no *neck* in this drawing, meaning that there is no distinct differentiation between reason (head) and feeling (body). The child has not developed much will power, that is he can offer little resistance to his own desires. The *hands* are proportionally well-drawn and turned outwards, meaning there is good contact with the outside world. The *genitals* are drawn normally for this age, meaning that the child is aware of his own sex. But the detailed 'private parts' could also mean that the child wets his bed.

The emphasis on the *shoes* indicates a fixed standpoint and is a sign of certainty. The shoes are rather large in relation to the rest of the body and there are cleats on the soles, which could indicate a certain aggression (fighting, kicking). Of course, it is also possible that the child has just received new soccer shoes, which is why he emphasizes them. Nevertheless it remains true that these shoes are especially good for kicking, and we wonder why they were given so much emphasis in the drawing (kicking a ball is a sublimated form of aggression that will be touched on later in this book in a discussion of aggression in children's drawings).

The *legs* are firmly planted on the ground, indicating that the child feels certain and earthed. The bodily proportions are adequate for the child's age; the child feels himself to be physically in balance. There are not many details in the clothes, which means that the personality has not yet become differentiated. The only detail in clothing is a *belt* as a dividing line between chest and stomach (and the genitalia) The belt that has to hold up and close the trousers (or the bladder?). The belt also indicates a division between feelings in the chest and in the stomach, meaning a distinction between superficial (the chest) and deeper (the stomach) emotions. No surroundings were drawn. That could be because the child did not have enough time to finish the drawing or because the outside world does not yet play a large role.

Conclusion
We can draw several conclusions from this drawing. It is about a boy who does not yet fully know what he can or what he wants. His intelligence seems normal. He has oral needs (sweets or sucking his thumb) and/or he is verbally aggressive. He has a lot of friends, but he also fights a lot. He does not pay much attention to what other people want or do. He likes to do as he pleases and does not listen well. He makes contacts

easily but he can become aggressive when angry. He is sometimes too childish for his age and acts like a clown. He is a thinker and he has imagination. He does not readily show his deepest feelings. There may be problems about his wetting the bed. As the youngest in the family, he may have to defend himself against his bigger brothers, and he may sometimes act like a clown to hide his anxiety.

Case illustration 2

A drawing by a ten-year-old boy. He goes to primary school and is intelligent, but others find his behaviour strange.

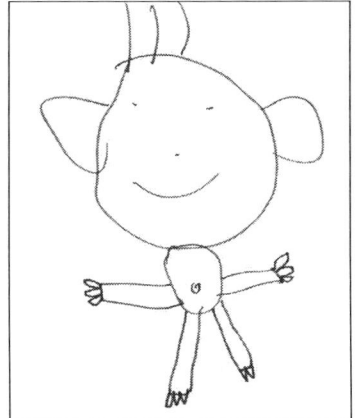

Drawing of a person (boy, 10 years old)

The *first impression* is that the drawing is childish for a ten-year-old boy.
The head is proportionally large and its relation to the body resembles that of a baby. There are three strands of hair standing upright, which indicates cognitive activity and strength. The ears are large, which indicates a conscience and the ability to listen to others. The arms and legs are drawn in almost the same way, as are the fingers and toes. The arms stretch outwards, which indicates good social contact, although there are only three fingers on each hand and they have the same shape as the toes. This could indicate an incomplete or disturbed body image. The legs are not on the ground, and there is little stability. There is no neck; the will is not well-developed. There are no clothes to underline the personality. A navel has been drawn on the abdomen, meaning that there is still a strong tie to the mother and that an independent ego has not yet been developed.

Conclusion

This drawing is more in line with a child of five and is too childish for a boy of ten. Because children (and adults), when feeling embarrassed or recalcitrant, sometimes draw matchstick figures in which there is little personal content, we may not immediately draw conclusions about the significance of this drawing. If, however, a child is unable to make a spontaneous (not copied) drawing of a person that has more details, we can certainly regard that as a signal.

The boy said that he had never before drawn such a good figure and that he was unable to do so.

It is known that the boy is highly gifted and has some autistic traits that are expressed in the drawing in the emphasis on the head and the strong lines as hair. There are no details in the head or body, and clothes and surroundings are absent or are drawn too childishly for his intelligence. His physical consciousness is underdeveloped, and, as a result, his awareness of his psyche and his emotions is also underdeveloped. For his age, he is too unaware of his body and his surroundings.

Having examined what is wrong in the drawing, we can now look at what is good. He has drawn a smiling mouth, which means that he has a positive image of himself. His conscience seems to be well-formed since the ears are in proportion to the head. His outstretched arms show possibilities of contact with the outside world and of making friends. His will is not well-developed, and this is necessary to overcome frustrations. However, there are signs that the ego and personality may grow because the abdomen with the navel and the four limbs show a tendency towards centralization.

Case illustration 3

A seven-year-old girl who recently moved and who feels somewhat insecure.

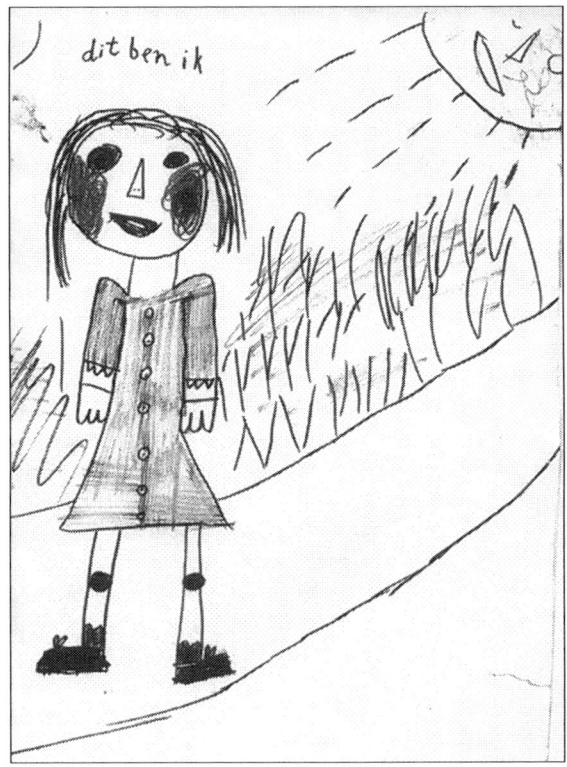

Drawing of a person (girl, seven years old)

The *cheeks* are emphasized: red cheeks are a sign of health but also of embarrassment (blushing). The *mouth* is slightly parted and the *lips* are emphasized, which could indicate special oral needs (thumb-sucking), emotionalism and sensitivity. The *hair* shows that the child knows she is a girl and accepts this fact. The *neck* is clearly drawn: there is a clear division between feelings and reason and the will is well developed. The *arms* have been drawn close to the body, indicating that it is difficult to make social contact; the *hands*, however, are clearly visible, indicating that contact is possible (if, for example, the other person comes closer). The *knees* are emphasized, which points to a certain stubbornness; it is also possible that the child has recently fallen *painfully* on her knees (Many accidents, such as falling or bumping into something, can also be cries for attention). The *shoes* have been drawn in proportion and indicate a strong base. The *legs* are spread, indicating that she is both relaxed (at ease) and certain (earthed). The *bodily proportions* are good and sufficient for her age.

There are seven buttons on the *clothes* (she is seven!) and decorations on the sleeves; the clothing is complete and highlights the personality. There is no division (no belt at the waist) between chest and abdomen, meaning that the deeper feelings from the stomach can flow freely to the surface at the chest and the other way around.

In the *surroundings* we see grass and sunlight, natural conditions. A road goes in an upwards direction from left to right, aiming towards the future and a higher ideal (the sun). The *sun* has a face and rays pointing at the child, which suggests the archetypal father in the presence of energy, warmth and light in the child's surroundings. The *words* above the head mean that the drawer wants to recognized or acknowledged.

Conclusion
This is a somewhat shy girl who perhaps enjoys sucking her thumb or eating sweets. She does not easily submit to someone else's will. She thinks before she reacts. She has some difficulty in making contact with others although she has a natural contact with the external world. She is intelligent and calm and has a stable base. She is sensitive and ambitious. She wants to be seen and heard.

In the final chapter of this book, further tips for systematically analyzing a drawing will be given.

CHAPTER 6

DRAWINGS OF HOUSES AND TREES

6.1 The symbolism of the house

A study of the drawings of houses and of trees shows us that there is again a universal development in the way in which houses and trees are drawn. And again, there are images with archetypal primitive feelings that we have inherited from our ancestors. In the drawings of both houses and trees, there is a visible relation between external reality and inner feelings that can be activated not only in children but also in adults. And we can again see that symbolizing an external reality is the creative source of the human psyche.

Starting at about the age of five, children begin to increasingly orient themselves to reality. The child draws what he or she knows, but there is still a great deal of room for the imagination and a drawing often tells a story. Houses and trees look a bit like the real thing but, at this age, they are still closely tied to universal and archetypal feelings. In other words, the symbolic significance of the house and the tree is important. In a later phase, children begin to adjust to reality and the standards and values that they learn at home and at school. From the seventh year, the child comes into what in developmental psychology is referred to as the 'latent phase', a point of rest after so many years of growth and learning. Nevertheless, children can (unfortunately!) still be taught at an early age to draw houses and trees according to the group standard, which can give rise to stereotypical drawings that have been learned and that do not come from the child himself. In a situation free from criticism or instruction, children draw people, houses or trees in original forms that come from the unconscious. Such a drawing is more valuable because the child has been given the chance to express his or her feelings. If there is someone who can understand something of the contents, the child might feel better understood.

Thanks in great part to a universal study by Rhoda Kellogg, we know that children throughout the world make the same sort of drawings of a house. In her book *Analyzing Children's Art*, Kellogg states that, 'The buildings or "houses" which children make are drawn alike all over the world' (page 123).

To understand the symbolic meaning of the drawing of a house, we must take various factors into account. We can examine a child's house in a variety of ways. We can look at the outside of the house: the type of house, such as a flat, a terraced house or a villa. These drawings of a house represent reality and they do not have a deeper psychological significance. The house where the child lives with his or her parents and possibly with brothers and sisters is the personal home in which more emotions are involved. And finally, the house can be seen as an expression of an archetypal feeling of protection derived from the archetypal mother, the factor who offers protection, care and nourishment.

The first time that a child experiences a feeling of protection and envelopment is during his or her time in the womb, the child's first 'home' that offered protection, nourishment and warmth. The womb was our first house and the circular opening of the vagina was the first entrance and exit. A house is also a place that can be entered and left again and that offers protection while we remain inside. In the development of a drawing of a house, we see that most children usually first drawing a round house with a round roof. They later draw a square house with a three-sided roof to which, in an even later phase, a door, windows and a chimney are added as the most important details.

The psychologist Jacqueline le Royer developed a 'Draw-A-House' test for children for her extensive study of this subject. She assigns great significance to the drawn house and its surroundings. She describes the house as 'various layers of the skin that envelops us: the mother's lap, the body, the family, the culture and the universe'. In her book *Traumbild Haus*, Ruth Amman, a psychotherapist (and a trained architect) and a teacher at the Jung Institute describes the house as *'Lebens-räume der Seele'*, the space where the soul can live. The house is where a child lives with his or her father and mother. The house represents a certain ambiance. In the child's own house, he finds protection, nourishment and peace because the people who live there love him. In the worst case, the house can be cold and unstable for a child, a place where he feels unwelcome.

A house has walls that form the boundary between inside and outside. The openings of the house are like the openings of the body: the door resembles the mouth and the windows resemble the eyes or ears. The door and windows often give a facial expression to a house.

1. The round house

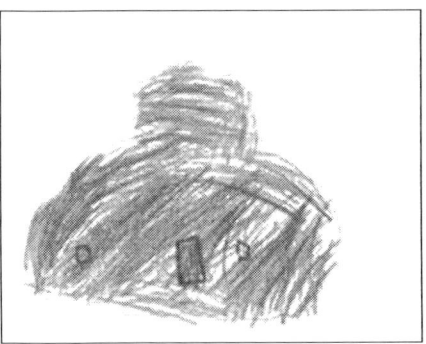

boy, five years old

If a child draws a round house, this is a symbol of the embryonic stage in which the house is thought of as the body of the mother. We often find round houses, huts or (Indian) tents among primitive people, and these round houses are usually built in a circle, just as in earlier days, cities were built from a middle point, a centre, with a strong wall as protection against the outside world. People felt protected in these round communities. In the child's first experience of protection, he or she is connected to – and is contained by – the mother. The child has not yet created his or her own place.

In therapeutic treatment, the word 'containing' is often used if the therapist wants to protect the child (a client or a patient) from impressions from the outside world. The child (client or patient) still has to grow and become independent before they can cope with the reality of the outside world.

2. The square house
The square house with its three-sided roof is the most well-known drawing of a house.
The Jungian analyst Ingrid Riedel points to the symbolism the square form that offers protection. The square house often has more personal traits, which will be discussed in detail here below.

A house is truly safe when it has a roof. The slanted or three-sided roof appears in all children's drawings, even in countries where this sort of roof is rarely found. This is because the triangle has a symbolic significance. The child is drawing not only a house with a slanted roof, but the child is also drawing *a square with a triangle on top of it*. The square is the symbol of protection, boundaries and stability, and the triangle is the symbol of the three-way relationship between father, mother and child. They represent important psychological experiences that belong together in childhood.

A lot of activity in the roof (the triangle) can indicate problems in the three-way relationship. The house that often has a facial expression is also connected to the roof. The roof can be seen as the upper part of the head, the brains, where the intellect is found and where thinking, remembering and dreaming take place. A lot of details in the roof cause a lot of activity in the head. This could the result of problems between the parents, forcing the child to keep a number of things in mind because the situation is incomprehensible.

3. Details of a house

The walls of a house provide support and stability and they separate the inside from the outside world. Behind the walls of a house are the secrets, possessions, good times, sex and tenderness of the inhabitants as well as their conflicts and arguments. Walls protect against threats from the outside. The sense of an inner and an outer world is experienced in a real house and depicted in drawings of a house. Expressing this can stimulate the still unconscious feeling of the psyche (the inner subjective world) and the psychological outside world (behaviour).

The *windows* of a house enable its inhabitants to look outside and those outside to look in. Curtains can be drawn or open and they add to a sense of safety and intimacy on the inside. Windows tell us something about the possibility of showing what is happening inside. When windows show light, it is easier to see what is taking place inside. Bars are sometimes set in windows to reinforce them and to prevent a forced entry (for example, in the world of emotions).

Round windows are common in children's drawings even though they are rather seldom in real house. These round windows often resemble eyes.

It may be that the child cannot yet draw square shapes, but square and round windows often appear in the same drawing. The round window could also signify a 'soul window', a round window known in many cultures through which the soul of a deceased inhabitant can leave the house. We could then assume that a round window was the soul of the house. The soul, the inner world and the Self are expressed in symbolic language as 'something round', and we can in fact say that each house has its own inner world. In the drawings of houses that follow below, we can find round windows, and the assumptions discussed here may prove applicable.

The *front door* of a house is very important because it is the place of transition from the intimacy of the house to the outside world. The front door is where someone can enter a house and can leave again. If a house does not have a door, contact will be difficult.

If the heating is on, there is warmth in a house, but it also must be possible to let the dangerous *smoke and fumes* escape. Steam is produced by cooking, meaning that the inner needs are being cared for. There is smoke coming out of a chimney if the house contains warmth and food. Smoke also means that a child can express himself by 'blowing off steam' and showing his inner feelings to the outside world.

4. The surroundings of a house

Looking at the surroundings of a house, we can see if there is a place to play and if there is contact with the outside world in the form of a road leading to the house. The surroundings tell us how the outside world is experienced, whether it is day or night, or what the weather is like. Most children add a sun, clouds, the moon, stars, etc. to their drawings of a house, and they draw fences, paths, people, animals, cars and roads that point to the relational elements.

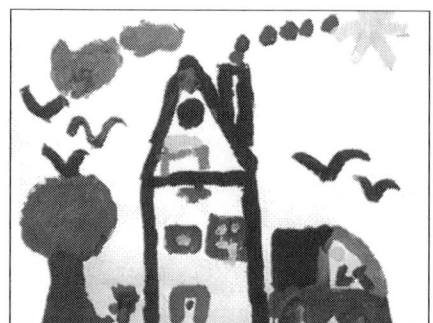
house with a tree, car, clouds and birds (boy, 8 years old)

If the *sun shines*, there is warmth and light in the *outside world*. The sun is often given a facial expression, such as laughing, looking angry, wearing sunglasses, having teeth, etc. The first drawings of the sun as described in drawings of sunrays made by toddlers and pre-school children do not have a face but they symbolize the feeling of protection from the outside world. When a facial expression is added to the sun, it indicates that there is a more differentiated feeling with regard to this protection.

Personifying heavenly bodies is in keeping with the previously described magical phase of children in which natural phenomena are given to human traits. The small child says that the sun is tired, the moon is going to sleep, etc., which is comparable to how our ancestors experienced natural phenomena as having divine traits.

The sun expresses the warmth and safety that the child experiences as the archetypal father, the figure who inspires action and provides light and warmth. The sun's facial expression shows us how the child experiences this figure. A laughing sun that cheerfully shines gives the drawing a positive aura. A sun that looks darkly (with sunglasses) may mean that it is looking critically or angrily. A biting sun (with teeth) may mean that the mouth is aggressive (with words). Sometimes, children colour the sun black, which makes it negative or even gloomy and oppressive.

The personification of the sun is an expression of the archetypal father, the figure who knows everything, is all-powerful, active and who forms the conscience. The archetypal father represents the strength that activates, a role that – depending on the roles in the modern family – may represent the personal father or the personal mother. But since the archetype of the father is a collective primitive feeling, the sun represents society, the school, friends, the church, God, etc.

Most children draw different facial expressions in the sun, just as they sometimes experience life (or their relationships with their parents) as happy and at other times as critical or dangerous, depending on the normal frustrations involved in childrearing. If the sun often or almost always has a negative expression, we may try to find out if the child experiences too many negative feelings in his or her daily life. These negative signals should not be labelled 'wrong' but should be seen as a healthy way for a child to express himself. We can follow a child's development if we remain aware of the meaning of a symbol and react adequately by, for example, offering encouragement, strength or comfort so that the child realizes he or she is understood and that someone can offer help.

A child soon draws *clouds* in the sky, meaning that the child feels the air around him and wants to make it visible. Children can colour light blue clouds or dark rain clouds, an indication of the atmosphere around the house. We can also look at where the clouds are in relation to the house or people. Clouds also mean that there is air to breathe. A dark cloud can bear down heavily on a house or a person. We can try to discover what the dark cloud is at that moment in the child's life.

Is there *vegetation* such as grass, trees, flowers and plants in and around the house? Vegetation is important for survival. It means that there are natural elements in and around the house. If there is grass and trees, there is also water (even if it is not drawn). Toddlers and pre-school children usually start drawing grass, flowers and animals before they draw a house since the child's first natural surroundings during the vegetative/animalistic phase are the most important (Neumann). The house is drawn at a later stage as people and the outside world (the collective) become more important.

There can be *fences, gates*, etc. around the house, indicating that the house is marked off as private property. Such signs of enclosures mean that the child can also mark himself or shut himself off. A house with a tall fence may mean that the child is part of a closed family that wants little contact with the outside world.

From about the age of seven, children begin to draw their houses more and more realistically. They usually do this from a *bird's-eye point of view*, from the rooftop. We can also look inside the house. Children find it important that everything is as it should be (according to the group standard) and they draw the rooms in detail with furniture and lamps, as if these were X-ray drawings. The somewhat inconsequent and varying perspectives are an expression of an exercise by the child to look at himself and his surroundings from another perspective.

If a child draws a human being (or a figure) next to the house, we can see the child in relation to the house. We may see a large house next to a small child or the other way around; this points to the child in relation to an adult at that moment. According to Royer, this points to a period in which the child has had to deal with the phases of omnipotence and submission. Either the child feels himself to be the master over the adult or the adult is the master over the child. In the (second) phase of stubbornness between the ages of five and six, the child can draw both situations almost simultaneously; he sometimes feels more powerful than the adult because he can get his own way or he feels powerless because he does not get what he wants.

A child sometimes draws two houses in one drawing. This is often the case when the child lives in two houses because the parents are divorced and each has his or her own house. Such a drawing sometimes enables us to see how the child experiences this situation. We can see how these two houses differ from each other. A drawing, however, is always a random indication. A child may have had a miserable weekend with one of the two parents and wants to express this in a drawing. At another time, completely different houses might be drawn. Although such drawings are not judicial evidence, they do indicate a certain feeling at a certain moment that the child wants to express. We should not use these drawings to trap a child because then he or she will no longer be able to or will want to draw. But we can try to solve any existing problems.

6.2 Learning to look at a drawing of a house

Case illustration 1

Two different girls drew the houses below.

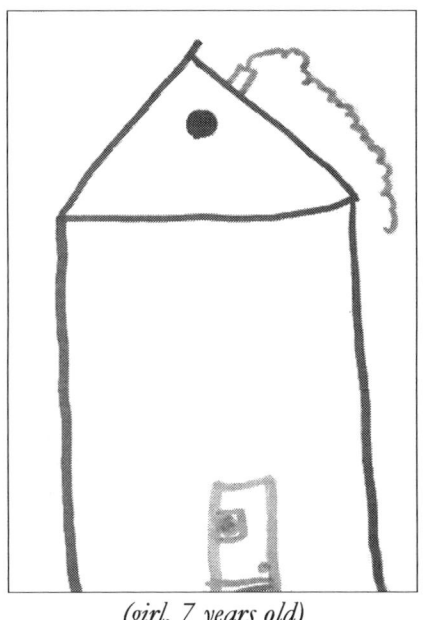 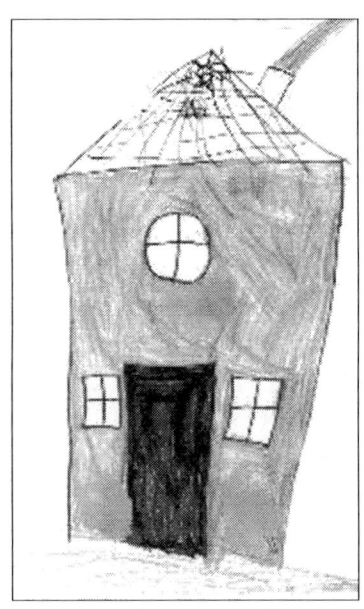

(girl, 7 years old)   *(girl, 8 years old)*

What are the differences?

The house on the left   **The house on the right**

Drawn at the bottom edge of the paper, which means that the parental house is still very important.	Is higher and on a diagonal line, which means that there is more distance from the parental home
The house has not been coloured, so there is a certain emptiness and blandness	The house has been coloured orange and the door is red. There is warmth and liveliness
The door has a window, a lock and a threshold so contact is wished for and possible, but it will be difficult	The door is large and heavy. It is clear where you have to be if you want to enter.

There are no windows. The inhabitant does not show her interior and does not let anyone look inside	The windows are large and secured with a cross. You can look inside and the inhabitant can look outside. There is still a certain amount of (self) protection
There is a 'soul window' in the roof, a round and dark window	There is a 'soul window' in the roof, a window that is open and protected.
The lines of the triangular roof are strong and clear, which points to a stable relationship between father-mother-child. The roof is otherwise empty except for the one dark window, which might indicate a feeling of loneliness.	The lines of the triangular roof are vague and interrupted. There are roof tiles and two round windows can vaguely be seen. The relationship father-mother-child is perhaps vague and chaotic. There is a great deal of action in the relationship and therefore a lot of activity in the mind.
The smoke from the chimney is curling downwards. This expresses feelings of warmth in the house, although it does not have much strength	The smoke from the chimney rises upwards (off the paper), which means that there is a firm channel for feelings and warmth.
The outer walls of the house are clear and strong, which means that the influence of the outside world cannot easily penetrate to the inside nor vice versa.	The outer walls of the house are interrupted and vaguely drawn, which means that the inside world may not be sufficiently protected.

Conclusion

The girl who drew the house on the left is shy, reserved and quiet. She speaks softly and perhaps sometimes cries silently. She has little contact with other children. She does not show her feelings. It is worthwhile to try to find out if there is something wrong with her or at her home.

The girl who drew the house on the right is self-assured, busy, extravert and active. The house makes a safe and protecting impression with evidently some extravert actions in the relationships between its inhabitants.

Case illustration 2

A nine-year old girl came to therapy because she was very active, she cried a lot and she had temper tantrums. At the first therapy session, she sat quietly at a table and did not want to talk very much. She also did not want to play. In fact, she really did not want to do anything. She said, 'I don't think I'll come back next week because I don't think this is helping'. Meanwhile, she began to draw on a piece of paper that 'just happened' to be lying on the table. She drew the house below

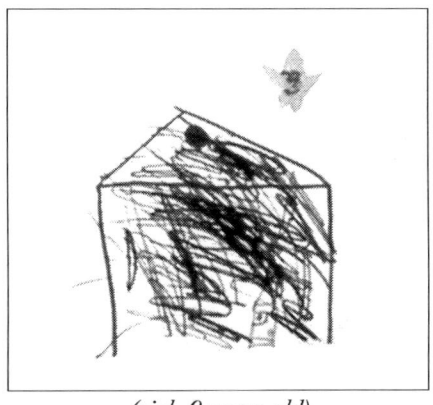

(girl, 9 years old)

The walls of the house were drawn with a dark purple felt marker and the door was drawn in pink. There is a narrow window drawn in black lines on the left and a purple circular window in the roof. She also scribbled black, red, yellow and greens lines in and across the house. The house was no longer there (or it had to disappear) and she scribbled across it without limitation. There is boundlessness in the house because she did not stay inside the lines of the drawing (just as in the first boundless drawings by children). The scribbles indicate a traumatic event in the house or they could point to a temper tantrum. The actual house, the home situation, and the archetypal house have been damaged; that is, the child's feelings with regard to safety and protection have been damaged. In the sky there is a yellow sun with dark eyes and eyebrows but it looks more like a star. It could be night and dark but the presence of a 'sunny star' might indicate a light in the outside world. A star is something that gives light and points the way, so perhaps there is someone who can help the child. The door gives access to the house and is fortunately visible. The child wants to and can be helped.

The girl remained in therapy and it was possible to speak with her parents about her home situation. The marriage was in difficulty and the parents wanted to have some time to think about counseling. In such a situation, the parents have to look for help because otherwise the child cannot be helped. In the worst case, the child can only be helped to become stronger so that she can endure the home situation.

6.3 The symbolism of the tree

Another example of a universal drawing is that of the tree. If a child can draw a house, he or she can usually also draw a tree. Both the house and the tree represent archetypal feelings. The first drawings of a tree, which often resemble a hand, have a straight trunk with a branch to the left and to the right and some short lines as leaves.

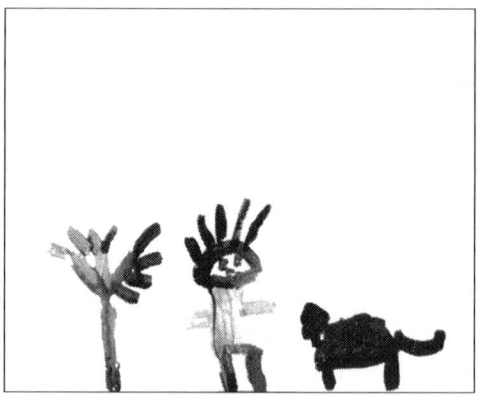

tree, person, dog (boy 5 years old)

Karl Koch is known for the tree test that he developed. Examining drawings of trees made by both children and adults, Koch draws important conclusions about the drawer's life and character development. Gisela Schmeer has investigated the therapeutic effects of drawing a tree and she gives examples of her interpretations in her book (*Heilende Bäume*). She demonstrates that drawings of trees often reveal something about the drawer's attitude towards life (constrained, open, free, hidden, stunted, empty, immature, one-sided, etc.). In her book *Maltherapie*, Ingrid Riedel gives an impressive example of how an anorexic patient saw herself reflected in the hollow and sick tree that she had drawn (p. 84). It is generally said that a drawing of a tree shows us something of the drawer's feelings about himself and that, by examining the form of the drawer's tree, conclusions can be drawn about the past, the present and the future as well as about the possibilities for further growth.

The tree has always been a symbol of life, a symbol not thought of by man but naturally present in man. This derives from the period when early man/our ancestral primates were able to escape danger in the primordial forests by climbing a tree. Primordial instincts lead the toddler to 'climb' into his or her mother's arms when danger threatens. The tree is probably one of the oldest symbols of life and survival in the history of mankind. The outline of a tree with a trunk and branches that spread in all directions makes it possible to represent the growth and descendents of a family in the form of the family tree.

Most psychological tests have found a correspondence between the way in which a tree is drawn and a person's attitude towards life. But these are just indications and impressions, not detailed analyses carrying judicial evidence about the present or about things that happened in the past. That is because unconscious and unknown factors always play a role (in the expression of a symbol) that we cannot yet see and that we cannot yet know.

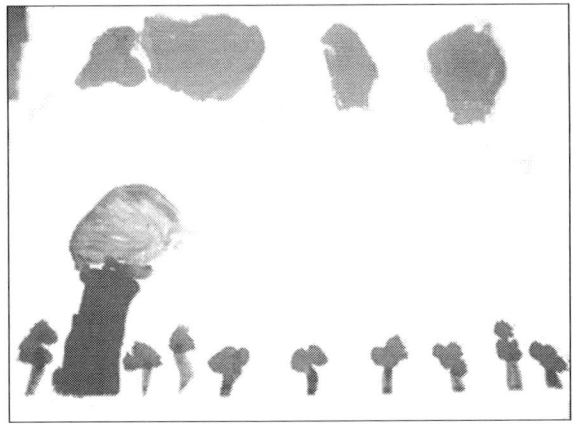

tree, flowers, clouds (boy, seven years old)

The tree is both a symbol of protection and of life. It is the archetypal tree, the universal, natural, human characteristic of strength, care, nurture and protection that every individual needs. A drawing of a tree shows us the extent to which this archetypal force is or was present in a child. A child can also draw a 'tree of wishes', so that the drawing works as a compensation. The child shows us what he needs and, to an extent, gives himself what he needs.

1. The trunk

We do not have to be a detective to see that all children emphasize the length of the trunk in their drawings of trees. The crown of leaves is proportionately small. We may assume from this that the child draws the tree as a personification of himself with the emphasis on growth in height. A child grows until he or she is between sixteen and eighteen years old; this is followed by ripeness and flowering, which may be seen as the result of the previous growth.

We could compare the length of the trunk with the years of a child's life. We sometimes see wounds in the trunk, and it is amazing to note how often traumatic experiences such as parting, moving house, etc. can be seen in abnormalities or wounds in the tree trunk.

The structure of the tree trunk also represents the physical contact with the mother (the tree as a mother symbol in which the child climbs when he or she looks for protection, as has been described above). There are various psychological layers in the significance of the trunk, and we can try to discover if there are connections between these layers. Take, for example, the smooth trunk which is difficult to get a grasp on and in which there are holes or wounds, or, in contrast to this, a rough trunk with a lot of structure that does offer a grasp even though there are wounds in the trunk.

2. Roots

In its natural form, a healthy tree needs a good system of roots. Psychological and therapeutic experience has shown that the roots of a tree in a drawing give an indication of the strength, anchoring and security felt in early childhood as well as the origin of life. Roots take nourishment from the earth and roots support the tree. From about the age of four or five, children are able to draw roots and to pay attention to them in their drawings. By looking at these roots, we can sometimes see what (psychological) nourishment a child gets (or needs) for his or her emotional life.

3. Animals

Animals are sometimes drawn in or near a tree. Animals in a tree are instincts that say something about desires and expectations. A bird in a nest, for example, means that an egg has been laid and that something is being hatched. It could also mean that the bird wants to leave the nest. Children sometimes draw an animal near a tree. The symbolic meaning of such an animal represents a certain aspect in the child's life and often in his or her character as well. It can be something helpful, such as a horse, but also something dangerous, such as a lion. A hole in the trunk may mean that, during a certain phase (during growth), the child needed a nest or a hole and that he or she missed protection.

4. Fruit
Some trees bear fruit, such as apples. If a child draws fruit in or near a tree, it often means that a certain situation in the child's life is 'bearing fruit'. It is a positive sign in the child's development.

6.4 Learning to look at a drawing of a tree
In a drawing of a tree, we look at various details, such as the roots, the trunk, the branches, the leaves and the surrounding. In addition, we must also keep in mind how children of a certain age draw a tree because, just as in the drawings of human figures, the form and the details of the tree follow a certain pattern of developmental psychology, both cognitively (knowing what a tree looks like) and emotionally (the tree as a symbol of certain feelings).

Case illustration 1

A seven-year-old girl went through a difficult period when she moved to another city two years ago.

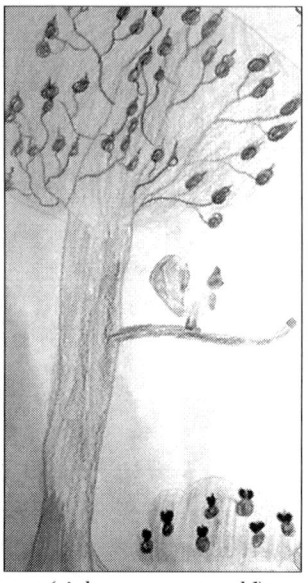

(girl, seven years old)

Here we see a tree with green leaves, many branches, (red) apples, a rough, brown trunk and strong roots. Seven apples are lying on the ground. A squirrel is sitting on a branch that juts out to the right. The trunk, leaves and apples have been drawn in proportion to one another, but the branch on which the squirrel is sitting does not match the rest of the tree very well. The trunk and the roots point to a healthy basis and development; there is good physical and psychological balance. The branch that suddenly juts out from the right may indicate a recent unexpected change. The little girl probably felt lonely and deserted during her move, and this is indicated by the squirrel. A squirrel is usually a shy animal that can provide for itself but has difficulty making contact with humans. But a squirrel is also a go-between (between the air and the earth) because it can climb up and down so quickly. In many cases, a squirrel can represent the feelings of a child who has difficulty in making contact and who feels as if he or she were floating between heaven and earth (or hell). Drawing (or playing with) an animal that represents such feelings helps the child to deal with these emotions. The squirrel is the child's friend. There is a positive attitude (which is symbolized by the fruit).

Case illustration 2

An eleven-year-old girl drew this tree after going through a difficult period. When she was three, she was placed in a foster home. Her foster parents divorced and, for the past year, she has lived with a new family.

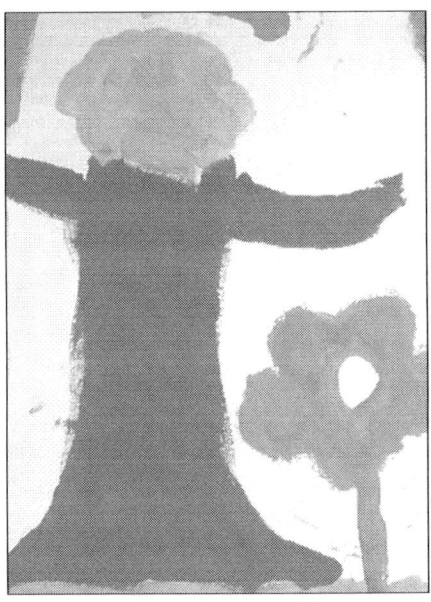

(girl, 11 years old)

This is an example of a tree that resembles a human figure. It could also be a woman in a long dress. There seems to be a relation between the tree and the flower. The tree is brown with green leaves and the flower is red and yellow. The tree might be making a gesture of embrace, but it also might be walking away. It might also be a woman who is dancing in a circle. Only the child who made the drawing knows the right answer. But the child might also say, 'It is just a tree'. The answer (or the significance) is not conscious and it is usually better not to ask any further questions or to confront the child with our own interpretations (referred to as 'containing' in therapeutic jargon). It is a hopeful sign that the flower has grown so tall by itself!

Case illustration 3

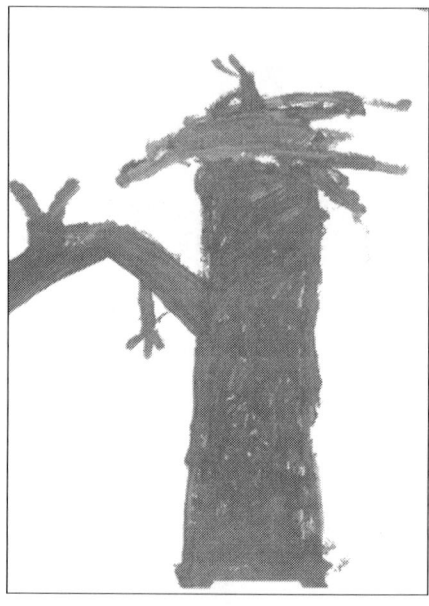

This tree was drawn by a seven-year-old boy.

The tree has a broken branch on the left as well as a hanging branch. There seems to be a rabbit sitting on the branch. The trunk is sturdy. The size of the leaves is in keeping with the boy's age, but they are strange because most children draw a round crown as foliage. Looking at this tree, you might wonder why there is such noticeable damage on the left side. The left side points to the past, the subconscious and the emotions (see also the discussion on space in chapter 9). Such an imbalanced tree could point to a trauma, a disruption, or at least to a wound in the child's emotional life. A tree such as this demands attention because something could be wrong.

CHAPTER 7

CHILDREN CAN DRAW EVERYTHING

7.1 The latency phase (7 to 10 years old)

At about the age of seven, children enter the latency phase. The term 'latency', meaning 'quiet' or 'hidden', is used to refer to this period in which not as many new developments occur as in the previous years or in the years of puberty yet to come. It is still possible to frighten children. They try to find an explanation for everything and they no longer take everything for granted.

The nine-year-old child who is told that Santa Claus no longer exists is psychologically capable of accepting this information as true. He or she has often already suspected as much, and the facts serve to confirm the feeling that 'something was not quite right'. The school child wants answers to questions and wants to know how the world works. What is electricity? Where does rain come from? Can I die? It seems as if the child is trying to obtain more certainty about the world around him, and the child's preferences for schedules, ordering things and rules should be seen as a search for and maintenance of a new sort of balance. The psyche's subconscious has been banished from the childlike paradise, and a new order has to be discovered by the intellect. Discovering the natural order of things leads to a simultaneous discovery of one's own nature.

A child of ten can differentiate between fantasy and reality. The developing child's natural possibilities for growth can then be used. The reality principle is prominent. The body is in proportion, which can also be seen in the drawings. This is the phase in which children can deal with possible conflicts or traumatic experiences from their infancy and earlier childhood.

Drawing is a pleasurable activity in this phase, and most children draw willingly and spontaneously. If a child gives a drawing away, this is a sign of contact. It is important to respond correctly, not by telling the child what is wrong with the drawing but perhaps by asking him or her to tell something about it. The child has gone through an important psychological phase of development that Freud referred to as the oedipal phase. The 'I' is now formed more by the difference between the sexes: 'I am a boy' or 'I am a girl'.

7.2   X-ray drawings

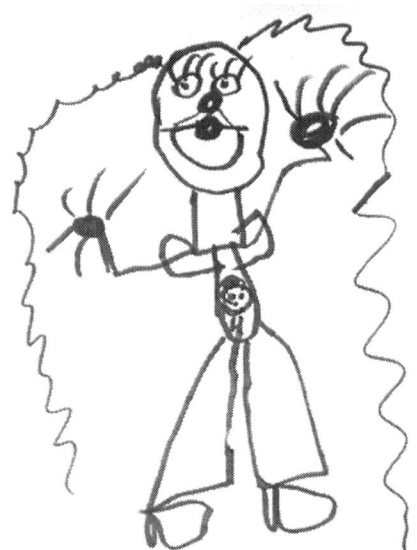

baby in the mother's belly (girl, 8 years old)

Children of seven or eight years of age draw what they know. They draw a baby in the mother's womb, chairs and lamps are drawn inside the windows of a house and presents are visible inside their wrappings. This is in keeping with the phase of wanting to learn and of trying to discover what lies behind things. They want to know how the world works and they ask questions about this. Intellectually, children are at the stage of 'fantasizing anticipation' (Piaget) or 'logical realism' (Luquet). They can imagine that there is something behind an object that they cannot see, such as the handle at the back of a cup. Children draw what they know and not what they see; their reality is intellectual rather than visual.

7.3 Drawings with a story

In these drawings, children experiment with perspectives, and we can see different perspectives in the same drawing (for example, looking down on to a scene in which things and people face forwards). This means that the child does not yet have an unambiguous image of the world around him and that various and contradictory viewpoints are possible.

In the history of art, we can find similarities to these drawings by school children. In paintings in the Middle Ages, it was normal to place the objects of the painting rather randomly on the canvas. In the painting 'Moses and the Burning Bush' (Nicolas Froment, 1457), there is a forest at the top of the painting where the Madonna and Child are sitting in a treetop; sitting below this is a man and an angel with a flock of sheep and there is a road leading to a town. In this same way, children between the ages of seven and ten 'narrate' their drawings. A story is told spread across the paper.

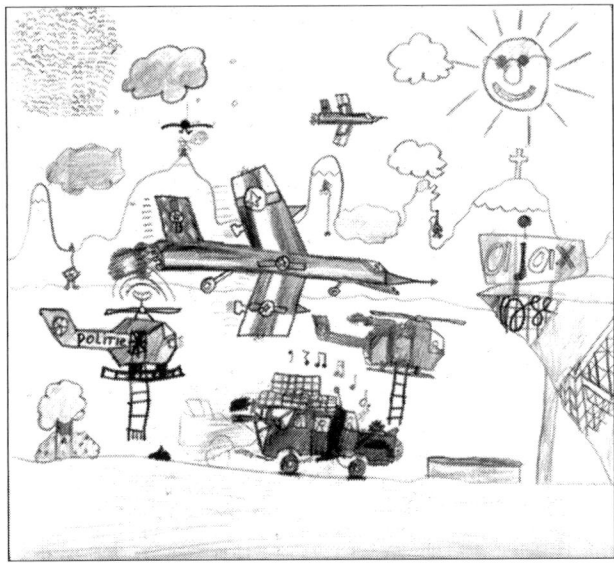

boy, ten years old

The above drawing tells this story:
There is a police helicopter with a rope ladder and a stretcher. And another helicopter that is hanging a rope ladder down to a sort of delivery van. The radio in this vehicle is very loud. There was first a trailer, but this did not belong (it was erased!). People are sitting in the car. A jet is flying above them and making a loud noise. There is

another airplane flying above the mountains. A man is climbing the mountain; he keeps falling off and hangs on a rope. The man on the other mountain is calling out something to a large bird. There is snow on the mountains and a cross at the summit of the mountain on the right. The sun is so strong that it has to wear sunglasses. Ajax is my soccer club. A large flock of birds is flying in from the left'.

This story could be a scene from a dream. The drawing contains a great deal of symbolism, the meaning of which would fill a book. We will return to the symbolic content in chapter 9 (*p.158*) when we discuss a case illustration that deals with the layout of a drawing. This drawing is included here now to show that children of this age can make narrative drawings.

We know from art history that perspective as we know it today was discovered only in about the fifteenth century. This is in keeping with intellectual development and the growth in knowledge of the natural sciences. People felt that the perspective had to be in line with the surroundings they saw, and they began to view their surroundings from another perspective. It seems as if the child repeats the history of this historical artistic development. The child first draws the symbolic and mythological phase (symbolic-religious painting), then adds people, animals, trees, houses and surroundings (paintings of landscapes, buildings and towns) and finally draws according to reality (the discovery of perspective). Having reached this last phase, the child has caught up with the present.

7.4 Cartoons and trick drawings

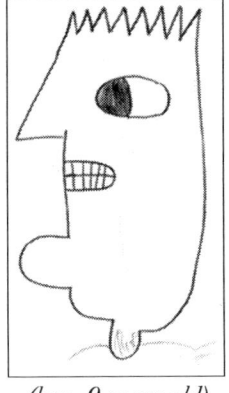

(boy, 9 years old)

Description: *a 4 and a backwards 5*

Between the ages of seven and ten, children often copy subjects and cartoon figures. They do not want to show off but they do want to make easy and 'pretty' drawings. Copying a drawing may also mean that a child wants to maintain control over a situation. Copying belongs to the phase in which children at school, in the street, during sports and at play learn standards and values from one another. This can also be seen when children play games with complicated rules with one another, such as marbles or trading cards. The value of a marble and the way in which the game must be played sometimes resemble the complicated rules of our tax system! Children learn from one another how things should be done, and it is difficult for adults to discover how these rules came into being. But children are able to follow the rules and agreements because winning and losing is done according to the rules of the game.

7.5 Spontaneous drawings

Although children of this age sometimes seem blocked in their ability to draw spontaneously, they are usually quite able to do so. Fantasy and reality work together harmoniously. It is important not to set rules about how the drawing should be done. It can be useful to see which children are artistically talented, but their self-criticism is usually not developed enough to stop them from drawing what they have in mind. They add more details, such as the sun, grass, birds, clouds, etc., to their drawings.

The child is well aware of the external world and is able to depict his or her surroundings.

7.6 The rainbow

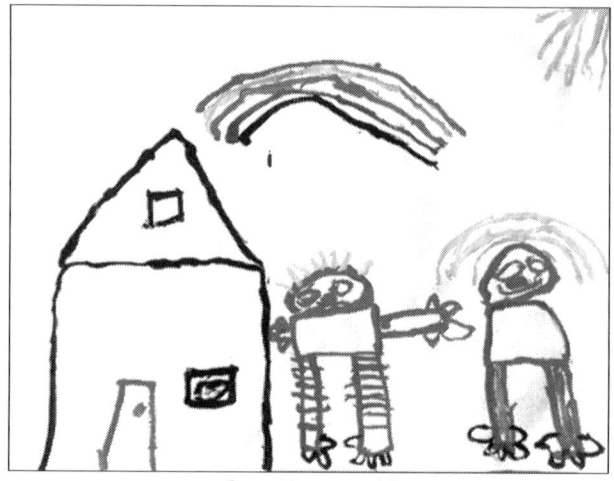

(boy, 7 years old)

Children often draw a colourful rainbow or a sort of umbrella above a person or a house. A rainbow appears after it has rained and the sun comes out again. This natural phenomenon is mentioned in all sorts of mythological and religious stories, where it signifies reconciliation between god(s) and man. Other myths and stories mention a treasure at the end of the rainbow, this being a sign of hope. If children draw a rainbow, it may mean that something has to be protected or that something must be reconciled (or was reconciled). It may also indicate some sadness in the child's surroundings and the child's hope for better things to come.

7.7 Traumatic events

School children may draw traumatic experiences; events that are too awful to imagine can be told by children in their drawings. Children sometimes also have an accompanying story to tell. Here again, the fear caused by an event can be somewhat controlled if the event is depicted. Moreover, the child can share his or her feelings with someone else; he or she has a sort of witness and no longer feels so alone. There have always been adults who have been able to help children in very difficult situations by stimulating creative expression.

One of the drawings on page one of this book was made by a nine-year-old boy from the United States. The terrorist attack by planes on the Twin Towers that caused so many people to spring from the windows must have made a tremendous impression on the boy. These images were repeated for days – perhaps even weeks – on television, a repetition that was evidently necessary for Americans to come to terms with the event. Reliving a traumatic experience in this way is a well-known psychotherapeutic method.

It is in the nature of children to take action. By making drawings about the attack, fear cannot settle. Using a form of expression (*ex* = out, *presse* = to throw) makes it possible to share the fear with the outside world. When that happens in a drawing, it is possible to talk about it with an adult: 'Yes, that's what it was like! It was terrible!'

Also well-know is the exhibit in Prague (adjacent to the Jewish cemetery) of drawings by Jewish children who had been imprisoned in the concentration camp Theresienstadt. These drawings express not only the daily misery but also the courage and hope felt by some of the children about their own fate or destination. Fear of the soldiers and everything they saw around them was movingly drawn. Both drawings and poems survived and have been published in Hana Valavkova's book *I Never Saw Another Butterfly*.

It is bad enough that, even today, children still have to experience war, misery and violence. The following drawing from 1999 was drawn by a girl from Macedonia, the war zone within former Yugoslavia. A journalist visited this zone and was given drawings by children who had seen and experienced terrible things. These drawings and the accompanying stories were published in a full-page article in the Dutch newspaper *NRC Handelsblad*. It is almost impossible to believe that children can make such narrative drawings. Some drawings speak of hope for a better future, as expressed in the butterfly that we often see in the drawings. A butterfly, as we know, is a symbol of metamorphosis, transformation and change. A caterpillar becomes a butterfly, and the butterfly lays an egg that becomes a caterpillar.

War Child, an organization devoted to the cause of children who have been through a war, has for years organized projects for children all over the world. Creative therapy such as music, drama, drawing and sports is used to help children deal with their war memories and war traumas. Creative therapists are contracted to supervise these projects and to train local care providers to help the children.

A child draws the war

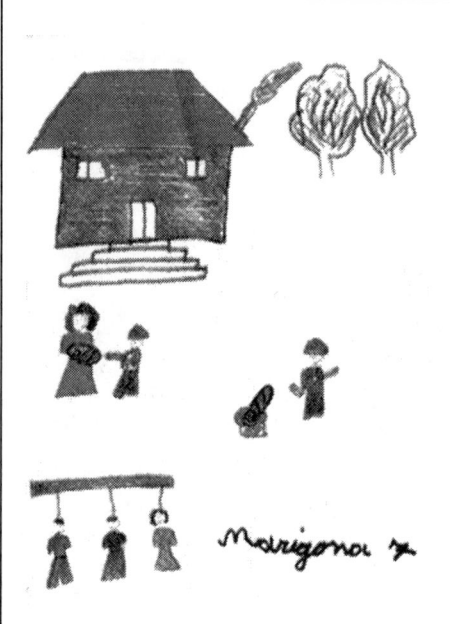

From: *NRC Handelsblad* 24 April 1999 (author: Cees Banning)
A drawing made by Marigona, a girl from Macedonia, during the war.
The accompanying text:
'This is our house. It is big. Behind the house there is a shed with papa's pigeons. I am allowed to feed them. Papa also has trophies because the pigeons can fly so fast. The police are shooting a baby because the baby's papa shoots policemen. The mother is sobbing. They also killed Azize's neighbour. I don't know why'.

Description and significance

This drawing by a girl from a war zone (with the accompanying text) needs no further explanation. The drawing is primarily in orange, red and green. There is no sun! The house is orange, the roof is red and the stairs are green. The people are wearing orange, red or brown/green clothes. The eyes of the house are wide-open 'in fear and anger'. The two trees in the background are green and orange, which makes them look as if they are on fire.

But these trees are the only form of vegetation and perhaps represent a form of safety and hope in the background. But green and orange are also the colours of soldiers wearing camouflage. Perhaps they protected the area and were witness to the entire scene.

At any rate, the child herself saw everything! Making this drawing will have helped the child to feel less afraid, as has been described above.

7.8   The period of group awareness

Boys and girls between the ages of eight and twelve withdraw into their own circle of contemporaries. In this phase, feelings of identity are expressed in group behaviour and group games. Boys express themselves in rough and tumble behaviour and they enjoy playing sports, outdoor games and competitive games. Girls tend to play more with each other and to play indoors; they enjoy handicrafts and caring for dolls and animals. On the one hand, the roles of boys and girls are physically determined but, on the other hand, their behaviour is even more determined by the way in which they solve problems: boys use force and action, girls consider the situation and are more socially oriented. Although this may seem stereotypical, we see this behaviour every day.

It is noteworthy that boys and girls of this age clearly prefer to spend their time with their own group. Boys have secret clubs and have a hut or a tree where they meet for exciting adventures. Girls have their best friends and they whisper and giggle with one another. Sexual differences are more defined in this phase. In the Western world, boys and girls discover and develop their own sex-specific characteristics and, partly thanks to the women's liberation movement, they are no longer so tied to traditional role patterns. Eventually, in puberty and later in adulthood, it will become clear to what extent there is a rapprochement and a harmony between the sexes.

Of course, not every boy's or girl's behaviour is so sexually specific at this age. There are girls who are tomboys and boys who act more like girls. Such a child is accepted by both groups and not considered strange. A personal sexual character will not be fully developed until after puberty. In this earlier phase, adult sexual preferences do not yet play a role, so that the child, if given the freedom, can playfully experiment with both roles.

The significance of the differences between the roles and the extent to which the roles are experienced have to a large extent been inherited over millions of years from our ancestor's experiences and instincts. It is good to realize that nowadays people are aware of these characteristics and that they no longer act on their instincts but rather take responsibilities for their actions.

The split between groups of men and women can be seen in the history of evolution. In primordial history, the role of the woman and mother was the most impressive. In primordial times, men and women (and male and female animals) lived separately. Children (and young animals) remained with their mothers until they were sent out of the home or nest. The females remained with the women and the males became independent. Evolutionarily speaking, the man had the task of finding a woman from families of another group. From earliest times men, having been sent away by (groups of) women, have had to learn to survive by working together and by fighting.

Primordial man saw that a woman bore children but he did not make any connection with his role in this process. As a result, women were all-powerful and terrifying because they evidently possessed powers of life and death. This determined the roles of women and men. Women cared for the children and the home, they gathered fruit and tilled the land while men went hunting and protected their territory. Both groups sought each other's support because this was necessary to accomplish their tasks.

Evidently, boys and girls still have to struggle, each in their own way, to break loose from the mother. At this age, they look for support from their contemporaries. The group, originally considered the enemy, now becomes a club of close friendships.

7.9 Drawings by boys and drawings by girls
Boys of this age are active and tough and they enjoy team sports and competitiveness. Male characteristics are explored and practiced. These 'young men' have to prove to their contemporaries and also to girls that they are courageous. Exploring (playing with fire) and going to forbidden places, especially those that are dangerous or prohibited, are among their

favourite activities. And at this age, they often need supervision or protection from an adult.

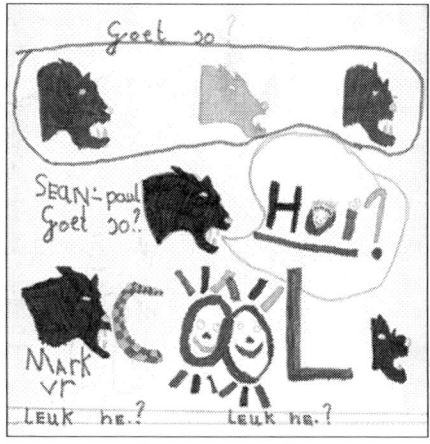
(boy, 9 years old)

In these drawings by boys, we often find active subjects and exciting adventures drawn with great enthusiasm. The archetypal male task of joining together to go on an adventure, discover the world and face all sorts of dangers is symbolically expressed here. In many mythological stories and fairy tales, the hero must fight a dragon or a monster in order to win the treasure. These stories show us that the developing person has to fight to free himself from a certain domination and has to learn not to be afraid. Children's fiction, TV series and computer games for this age group often involve these sorts of exciting and adventurous subjects: a secret treasure map, dangers that have to be faced and the villain who has to be captured by the young detectives.

Girls of this same age also draw specific subjects. At this age, they often draw a social situation in or around the house. They also draw animals, such as horses and cats, animals that exist and that they actually care for, brush and pet. In this way, they practice the archetypal female task of nurturing and protecting. They enjoy reading books about girlfriends and the adventures of girls' clubs, about girls who have a special friendship with a horse, or about a horse that saves someone's life. In many fairy tales, the horse is the guide for a young woman (or man) who is going to another country or surroundings.

They often encounter difficulties along the way, and the horse often knows which road to take or how to solve a problem.

In myths, the horse is regarded as being clairvoyant and having hidden strengths (Pegasus) and in fairy tales the horse helps the child to reach his or her destination (Grimm's *The Goose Girl*).

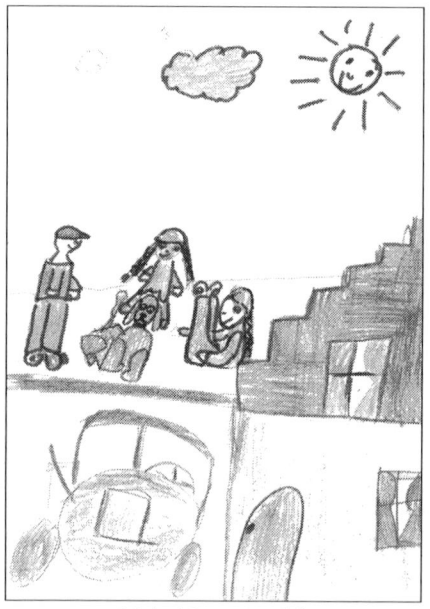

(girl, 10 years old)

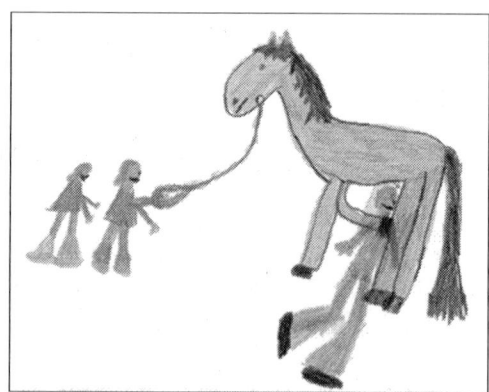

(girl, 10 years old)

7.10   Drawings of boats

Both boys and girls of this age often draw a boat, a steamship, a submarine or a sailboat. The boat represents the voyage of discovery to an unknown world.

It is worth pointing out that girls more often draw a sailboat (that sails under its own power with the wind), whereas boys more often draw a steamship or a submarine (that involves more technical power).

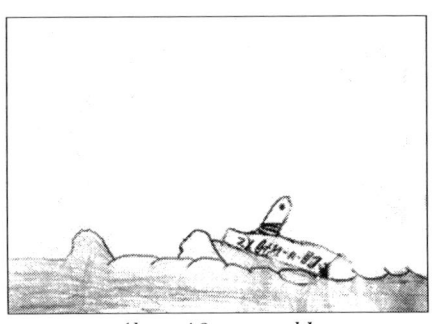
(*boy, 10 years old*)

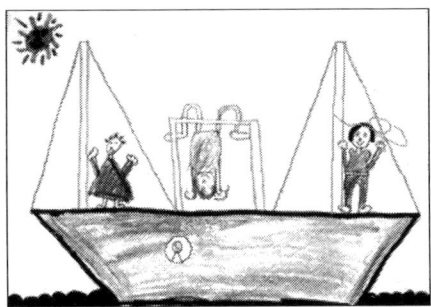
(*girl, 10 years old*)

Both sexes show that they are on their way to explore the world; they are practicing for the coming period of puberty in which the child has to become independent of his or her parents and leave the old world of childhood behind in order to become a self-sufficient adult.

The journey to adulthood by boat can be found in the ancient myth *The Odyssey* in which the hero Odysseus has to leave his beloved Penelope and sail wherever the winds take him. He is shipwrecked, has to do combat and is tempted by sirens before being reunited with his beloved. Psychologically, this epic describes the courage that a person needs to withstand tribulations, overcome fears and keep faith in his final destiny (Eva Sigg, *Penelope und Odysseus*). This is yet another example of human development being based on archetypal strengths and experiences. The archetype in this case is the explorer who time and again spontaneously reveals himself to mankind.

The child who fantasizes about distant voyages and about discovering new worlds as an explorer is at that moment connected to the archetype Odysseus. The child who must wait until Odysseus returns from his travels is at that moment connected to the archetype Penelope, who had to bide her time and go through a process of maturing. Of course, not every boy identifies with Odysseus just as not every girl identifies with Penelope. Both archetypes play a role in both boys and girls because they concern basic feelings that are universally human. It may be that one boy or girl feels more attracted to Odysseus while another feels more attracted to Penelope. Friendships between children with opposite archetypal preferences may result in both sides learning from each other. Odysseus and Penelope represent universal human feelings that are still valid today, namely that young people must free themselves from the 'mother's island' and go off in search of their own world. As we have seen many times already, archetypal content and mythological stories have been modernized so that they can be told again and again.

7.11   Aggression in children's drawings

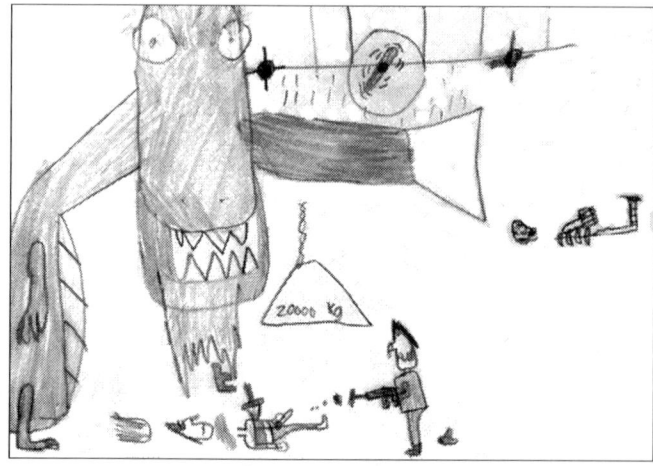

(boy, 9 years old)

Aggression may be prominent in drawings made by this age group, especially in drawings made by boys. We must learn to see the significance of such drawings from the perspective of the child's situation. For example, a child who makes a drawing of people fighting or of victims and wrongdoers may be depicting his or her own aggression but may also be expressing fights at home or at school. Fights, wars, victims and wrongdoers may also express a fear of the aggression that the child sees in the adult world with its wars and violence on television and in the newspapers. Aggression in drawings can also be an expression of anger that the child cannot express in his or her behaviour. For example, a child who withdraws into himself because he is teased at school can show enormous aggression in a drawing, thus expressing the anger that he feels internally. An aggressive drawing is a signal that we should not interpret too quickly. The drawing makes us aware of the situation and we can help the child by saying, 'I see someone in trouble' or 'That situation looks very dangerous'. The child must then decide if he or she wants to explain what the aggression in the drawing means.

What is true of drawings can also be seen in children's games. If children choose to play war games, this is often seen as a reflection of war situations in the world of adults, who sometimes forbid children to play with these sorts of toys. But it should not be forgotten that war games among children have nothing to do with war and violence in the adult world of political power struggles. If a child is forbidden to fight in a game or to play at being a hero, he or she can never practise fighting for a just cause. In a fight, a child can experience the fact that there are two sides involved and that a choice must be made between good and bad. If a child attacks other children when playing because he or she feels powerless or afraid, it is better to let the child play with toy soldiers so that the child learns to choose the side of what is good. This enables the child to differentiate between good and bad, and he can use his aggression to fight for a good cause, such as protecting the weak, demanding justice, becoming a top athlete or earning a diploma. Fury, fear and anger are no longer equated with bad, and the child learns by playing these games that these feelings also lead to being good and strong. The child who is told that he or she has to be nice but who is expected to fight to achieve a goal will be confused. It is better to pretend to fight or to go to war in games than to have children express their aggression only in sports. If we forbid a child to express inner feelings in games because we are afraid that the child is imitating the adult world, then we are judging the child by adult standards. And we fail to give the child the opportunity to overcome any future difficulties by fighting the good fight with fair play and fair rules.

It is, of course, completely different if children behave aggressively and trespass the rules of the game by acting as adult soldiers or even murderers. These children have probably never learned to play and should be helped to learn to do so. The question is not how this should be done but that it should be done (see Robert Bly, *Iron John; A Book about Men*).

7.12 Depression in children's drawings

When we see a drawing with little action or one in which almost nothing seems to be happening, we quickly assume that the child must be very quiet and perhaps even depressed. But here again we should not rush into making a judgment. A quiet or empty drawing may reflect a child's feeling of emptiness but it can also be a sign of inner peace. It is also possible that the child draws the peace he or she needs in a noisy world, in which case the drawing is a wish for peace and quiet. When looking at a drawing, we can note the facts (for example, there is little activity in a drawing), but then we have to examine what these facts mean in the unique case of the individual child. We should beware of making a rash judgment and should always take into account the personal circumstances of the child who made the drawing.

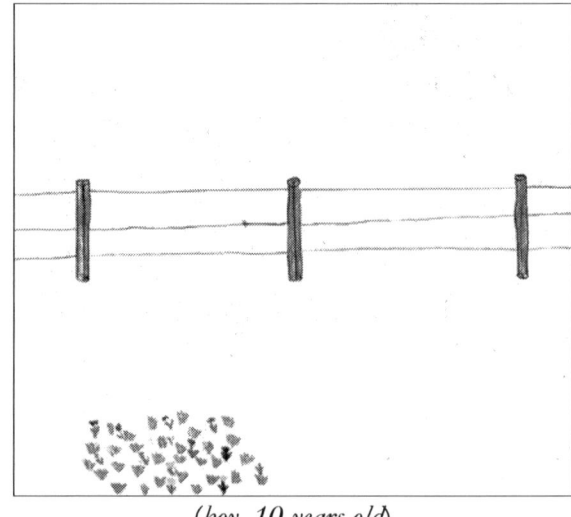

(boy, 10 years old)

Description

A barbed-wire fence. In the foreground, red and light green flowers.

Significance

This drawing makes a quiet and somewhat strange impression for a boy of ten. There is certainly some sort of limitation or closure. The small leaves in the foreground (green and red) are a sign of hope and life. There is barbed wire, but the presence of that early spring green growing upwards is a healthy sign of life and hope.

CHAPTER 8

ADOLESCENTS DRAW THEIR OWN LINES

8.1 Puberty (10-15 years)

Puberty is the period of transition from childhood to adulthood, a transition that begins for some children as early as ten years old when both biological and psychological processes of maturing begin to play a role. Children may be emotionally confused or restless. They project their criticism of themselves (physical or intellectual) onto the external world; the adolescent often complains that everyone else is stupid and ugly and that they just do not understand or they think it is a waste of time to try to talk with others, especially with their parents. What the adolescent is actually thinking is 'I'm stupid and ugly, I don't understand myself and I don't know how to communicate with others'. We will see that drawings made by adolescents express these specific feelings that accompany adolescent development. Adolescence is characterized by feelings of confusion, loneliness, idealism, romance and searching for one's own way. As we will see, the healing art of artistic expression is present in this group of young people and is needed in their process of becoming conscious and mature. Expressing feelings in all sorts of non-verbal rituals, such as music, dance and other forms of artistic expression, is necessary in order to deal with this phase of development.

It is the task of the adults to protect and guide adolescents in this important transitional phase by giving significance to their rituals of transition, creating circumstances where these rituals can safely take place and giving young people the opportunity to express their feelings creatively.

In this phase, the adolescent is again going to question who and what he or she is and how he or she wants to deal with his or her environment. It is the adolescent's task to free himself from his parents in order to become independent and adult. And as the adolescent becomes independent, he will look differently at his parents or guardians.

The development of the adolescent phase has been extensively dealt with in international literature. A well-known study is *'The Handbook of Clinical Research and Practice with Adolescents'* by Patrick H. Tolan in which the adolescent's biological, cognitive, moral, psycho-social and psycho-sexual development is described. Problems and Interventions are discussed in the last part of this handbook. This study demonstrates that, just as in childhood, there are universal experiences and developments in adolescence. Of course, however, the time, place and circumstances in which a child – and a adolescent – grows up influence the development of his or her personality.

In puberty we again see the connection with our predecessors and our evolutionary history. Here again is the struggle to become independent and responsible for one's own life and the ever-recurring task of the new generation to be innovative. Here too we see that man again discovers something that has always been present: becoming conscious of the human status so that a person is created who feels responsible for his deeds and actions. The adolescent who has to take leave of his childhood and join the world of adults goes through a process of becoming independent that can be compared with the process of being born. The adolescent has to leave the ideal situation of 'how it used to be' and to fall outside this world into the cold and unprotected world of adulthood. The mother (and the father) knows that the child has to leave, and the child knows that he or she has to leave the mother, just as during birth. This second birth is natural and inevitable, but that does not mean that it is always without pain or dangers. The child has to leave because he or she otherwise hangs between a child and an adult and remains a dreamy, childlike or irresponsible personality.

Parents can recognize and empathize with this development. They can support their children if they understand the true background behind adolescent behaviour. They probably once went through the same process of freeing themselves from their parents. If, when younger, parents did not or could not go through this process successfully, they may still tend to act like adolescents, which is always very confusing for the real adolescents. Parents must realize that they have to let go of their adolescent children. They may feel powerless when their child dismisses everything and everyone as being worthless. They should not regard their (temporarily bad) relationship with their child as a personal failure but as a sign that the child is going to free himself from the parents because that is how things should be (Kiepenheuer, '*Crossing the Bridge, A Jungian Approach to the Adolescence*').

But even the well-behaved adolescent who obeys and sometimes even idealizes his parents may be cutting himself short. A delayed adolescence always involves more pain and struggle. Changes in the psyche may occur in the period of physical changes during puberty. If these changes are not fully effected in puberty, then puberty may have to be experienced again later in life. This is a reason for parents to ask the adolescent and themselves what is causing the stagnation.

8.2   Rituals of transition

The developments in puberty are an archetypal necessity, the collective human primordial characteristics that all humans have experienced and will experience at all times and in all cultures. Roughly speaking, the development of the child that has to free himself from the protection of the parental family and the nurturing mother can be compared with man's evolutionary struggle to free himself from unconscious nature. It is the conscious man who has to step forth out of the paradise of childhood ('Mother' Earth) to create his own life.

Among primitive peoples, becoming free from the mother's care was always more difficult for boys than for girls. The rituals of transition for boys were performed by the adult males and, afterwards, the young man could never return to the women's circle. The rituals of transition from a girl to a young woman were more physical and natural because they usually happened when menstruation began. But for both sexes the rituals were the same in that the young people were taken from their families and made to undergo painful and frightening rituals. They were left by themselves and had to survive. They were often given a new name and, when they returned to their families, they had a new status: as if they had been born again. In some rituals, the young people had to scream at and even ill-treat the parents (the Papuans). The rituals of transition were supported and performed by the community, which consisted of the parents and the community's wise men and women.

Adolescents today are also introduced to a new world, not in the same way as their predecessors, but in keeping with the prevailing means and circumstances.

8.3 Contemporary rituals

For decades, religious communities and academic social clubs helped to guide young men and women to adulthood. Christian or Judean groups usually prepared these young people for a godly life in which the rights and duties of marriage were taught. Some academic clubs, which were only for the rich, had initiation rituals that were rather dangerous. In addition, compulsory military service was used in many countries as a means of initiating young men. Nowadays, however, religions, universities and the military play a smaller role in guiding people to adulthood. Old rituals of transition have disappeared in many parts of the world because they no longer fit in with this period of liberalization and emancipation.

There is, however, a sort of ritual today in the form of teachers who go camping with young people between the ages of ten and fifteen. These school camps have been organized for decades in almost every European country as well as the United States and Japan. In these school camps or another sort of youth camp (for example, organized by Scouting or soccer clubs), adolescents can experience the adolescent transition in a meaningful ritual. Usually, the supervisors, naturally aware of the unconscious but archetypal need of these school children, are able to create a programme that meets the primordial demands of the adolescent's rituals of transition. The popular school camps have programmes and activities that can be compared with the old rituals described above that we also see among primitive people. And these young campers often pitch their primitive tents in places completely removed from the protection of the parents, where they have to learn to survive under the guidance of the old and wise teachers. They camp in the forests in huts or tents, they often have to cook their own food, they are assigned tasks and duties, there is a frightening nocturnal scavenger hunt, competitive games, trials of strength and chances to enjoy new outdoor experiences (canoeing, climbing, making campfires, hang-gliding, etc.). The difference between these rituals and those from earlier times is that boys and girls almost always experience these rituals together rather than in separate groups. This is in keeping with modern man's growth of consciousness and emancipation, processes in which personal female and male characteristics receive less emphasis and in which universal human characteristics with both female and male characteristics are increasingly experienced and accepted.

8.4   Music and dance in puberty

Music plays a very special role in the world of adolescents and young people. Whether it is house, gabber or rock music from the 1990s, the twist and rock-and-roll from the 1950s and 60s or the waltz and the tango from the 1920s, all of these music and dance combinations can be traced back to the old, primordial sounds, rhythmic dances and rituals of transition of primitive man. Pop music, especially in and after the period of the Beatles, gained widespread attention not only because it was new and popular but because the texts were about subjects that interested young people. In the 1990s, Madonna became a symbol of emancipation for girls, so that the typically sweet side of the young virgin was replaced by the image of the temptress and the witch. Boys admired Elvis Presley, 'the King', and the rock star Prince. Here again we see the archetypal figures (dating from the collective unconscious) of the mother (madonna), the king and the prince!

The music and the texts criticized the old values and asked new questions about the meaning of life. With intoxicating pills and hypnotizing rhythms, young people sought to expand the borders of consciousness. This same phenomenon is known in tribal dances among primitive peoples when the dancers fall into a trance after repeatedly making the same dancing movements in the same rhythm. Primitive man did this to gather courage before a battle, just as today's adolescent does. The courage needed to go their own way and discover their own beauty and strength. If an adolescent becomes trapped in the ecstasy (xtc!) of drugs and alcohol, he or she cannot become combative and will remain discouraged and dependent. Young people who do not have the opportunity to give form to this search for their own identities and the transition to adulthood under trustworthy supervision often use drugs or alcohol to excess in order to stay in their trance. This unsatisfied desire leads to a weakening and collapse of the personality.

We can also see the rituals of transition in the mythological stories such as those involving the figure of Dionysus. These stories tell of wild ceremonies that were held in the forest. Dionysus signifies experiencing passion and the animal godliness of the soul. Psychologically, Dionysus is the power that alters the status quo; wherever he goes, there is creativity and things change. He symbolizes dynamism, excess and intemperance. On the one hand, there is ecstasy and, on the other hand, terror and the fear of death. These are again archetypal feelings that, if their deeper significance remains unknown, can have a negative influence on man's psyche. If the archetype is recognized and both the positive and negative sides are allowed, then these primordial needs can be attended to during puberty.

The old folk dances that were once – and sometimes still are – danced by boys and girls, that involved attraction and repulsion and that allowed people to display their beauty, strength and endurance are similar to the modern Western dance movements of today's youth in discos, clubs and at school parties. Throughout the ages, dance rituals have been altered or suppressed by religious and cultural authorities, but whether we look at the nineteenth-century quadrille or the twentieth-century hip-hop, we see that all of these dances are performed by men and women in an attempt to get to know one another better, to flirt and to experience feelings of ecstasy.

8.5 Problems in puberty

In cultures in which religion has lost its authority, where young people are not connected to a school and where there are few wise old men and women left, we see that young people often go in search of substitute leaders. These can be political or religious groups, sects, gangs or even idols and superficial trendsetters.

The transition from childhood to puberty has always been a painful one and today's adolescent still experiences this transition as difficult and painful. Today, it is not so much that the fourteen or fifteen year old has to leave the parental home, but that the adolescent has to free himself from the habits and rules of his own 'inner house'. This inwardly felt archetypal and universal task leads to feelings of fear. If the adolescent does not recognize this fear – if he does not learn to shudder – he cannot truly become an adult and he will not develop any empathy for others. This is the theme of the Grimm fairy tale *The Story of a Youth Who Went Forth to Learn What Fear Was*, in which a young man did not learn to shudder. In her book *Wege aus Angst und Symbiose, Märchen psychologisch gedeutet*, Verena Kast discusses the significance of this fairy tale. A young man is put into all sorts of situations that would terrify others, but he shows no fear.

In puberty, a boy first becomes aware of the female and emotional sides of himself. Only then can he feel empathy for others. A girl has to discover male characteristics in herself, such as being active and daring to be independent. These contradictory feelings have to be integrated. Risks have to be taken and this will cause fear as the boy or girl begins to doubt whether he or she wants to make the transition to adulthood.

Today's adolescents have to be convinced that their life of ease at their mother's side has ended. Mothers have to let their children go and fathers have to act as wise men for these children. All of the parties involved have a task. If one of the parties does not fulfil his or her task, there will be problems resulting in a lack of feelings of physical vulnerability (senseless violence, self-mutilation, aggression), depression (skipping school, using drugs, excessive drinking) or a feeling of grandeur (drug dealers, big spenders, excessive attention to one's appearance or clothes). Young people look for an escape from the parental home in clubs, groups and like-minded contemporaries. Although these groups of adolescents are often considered difficult, this phase of life is the most interesting because ideals and expectations being formed by young people are based on a natural inner impulse. If adolescents do not have the opportunity to experience this phase meaningfully, they run the risk of finding themselves in a crisis. If the adolescent gives up trying to look for the answer to the meaning of life – with the consequence that the answer will then never be found – he or she can become apathetic or depressed or can continue to act like an adolescent for the rest of his or her life (Kiepenheuer, *Crossing the Bridge*). Puberty is not just a certain phase of life but especially a phase of change, of great changes at the physical level and equally as great in the psyche. In the previous chapters, we saw how much the psyche was influenced by bodily changes, and we can imagine how much the psyche is influenced by the intense bodily changes in puberty. Parents should understand that it is the adolescent's task to implement changes for the new generation. The difficult task for the parents is to release the child while also offering protection.

As already discussed, inner experiences (of the psyche) are expressed in external (material) form. These healing-art mechanisms also play a role during puberty, especially in music, dance and rituals, but also in expressive art forms, such as drawing.

8.6   Drawing in puberty

After going to primary school, adolescents go to a secondary school that usually offers art classes in which pupils are given a mark for their work. Because adolescents are so critical of themselves, they may not enjoy drawing spontaneously since they think that they cannot draw (well enough). Nevertheless, it is good if the adolescent can find a way to express his or her feelings in this phase. Music, dance, or writing stories or poems can all be healing arts for this age group. If a drawing assignment falls into the world corresponding with the development of the adolescent's psyche, he or she will work on it with pleasure. Below are some examples of subjects that are in keeping with puberty.

1. A new perspective

Because the adolescent's perspective of the world around him has changed, this will also be reflected in his drawings. Both boys and girls usually enjoy drawings in which they may experiment with perspective. The graphic designer M.C. Escher made drawings with impossible perspectives, such as the well-known *Waterfall* in which the water cascades down and flows up at the same time. Such an impossible perspective gives adolescents the opportunity to play with their future possibilities.

It is worth noting that Escher, who lived from 1889 to 1972, made great use of mathematics, rhythm and music in his drawings. Escher wrote that *'..when, drawing on paper or engraving in wood, the hand makes repeated rhythmic movements as in a dance, when the artist feels the urge to emphasize with his voice, by singing.'* (M.C. Escher Life and Work, p.174).

This is a good example of a drawing assignment that teachers (and therapists) could give to adolescents in a classroom situation. It almost seems that Escher's mathematical drawings were the forerunners of today's computer drawings in which mathematical drawings can easily be made in all sorts of colours and forms.

2. Fantastic and surrealistic

Dream images, architectural structures that improve the world, heroes, fighters for a good cause, science fiction subjects, etc. all belong to this phase of life. And we often see drawings that belong to the way in which adolescents think. They are looking for a better world, they think they can change the world and are in search of answers to the world's problems. Drawings of a utopia or an ideal world are the result. Surrealistic drawings (such as those by Dali) may be made to express the alienation felt by the adolescent when he realizes that the old world has disappeared and the new world cannot yet be trusted.

3. Cartoons

Copying drawings, cartoon figures and cartoons – rather than making spontaneous and original drawings – may be seen as an attempt to stay in control of a situation and to hide one's own uncertainty or feelings. It is only logical that adolescents are insecure for a time, and it is healthy if they have found a form of expression that allows them to retain control. But in their cartoons and the accompanying texts, adolescents can depict themselves and the world around them in a very creative and original way, often by putting things into perspective or making fun of things.

4. Black and white drawings

Black and white drawings as an expression of black and white thinking are also in keeping with this age group. The colour black is also appropriate for puberty. In this phase, the adolescent experiences intense feelings but, not knowing how to deal with them, he represses them. Clothes are black, behaviour is sober and negative and drawings lack colour.

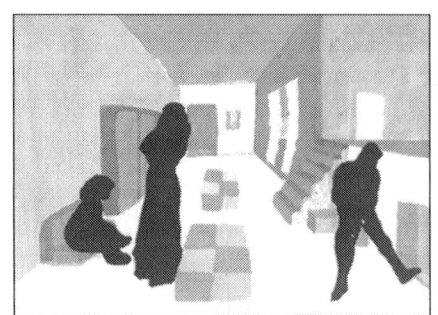
(girl, 13 years old) 'Perspective'

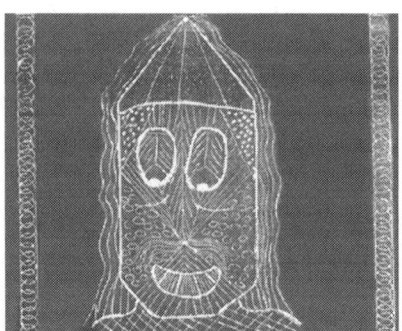
(boy, 13 years old) 'Graffito'

Using the colour black may be a healthy attempt to repress feelings (the colours) and to gradually let them reappear in a later phase. The technique of 'graffito' is very apt here: an underlying layer of various colours drawn in crayon is covered by a layer of black paint. When the paint is scraped away, the colours again become visible.

5 Drawing with feeling

In puberty we often see drawings in which feeling of love are expressed, romantic drawings that depict relationships with romance and fantasy. In drawings of humans, an idealized image, such as film stars, fashion models and impressive figures from cartoon strips, is often drawn as a object of identification. We also see drawings that depict loneliness in an empty landscape, a lone wolf, a prostrate human, etc.

8.7   Children's drawings on the World Wide Web

Good examples of children's drawings can be found on the Internet, where parents and children can nowadays easily place a drawing on a website. As a result, we are able to view all sorts of drawings made by children around the world. Examples of such a websites are: *the Australian Worldwide Kids Art Gallery* www.theartgallery.com.au/kids art.html. (2004) and www.childrens-drawings.com/eng/museum.htm (*The international Environmental Children's Drawings Contest* (2006) .

Here we can find diverse sorts of drawings that have already been discussed in this chapter and drawings that will be discussed later in this book. From tadpoles to trees, houses, animals, fantasy figures and drawings typical of an adolescent. The drawings come from Australia, the USA, Russia, Iran, England, India, etc. These are wonderful examples for the readers of this book to examine to see if they can discover the universal forms and subjects that we have been discussing. What is missing is the first series of scribbles (the boundless drawing, the spirals, crosses and balloons). That is understandable since, as we have already explained, most parents do not understand the significance of such drawings and regard them merely as doodles.

8.8   Giving up drawing

Adolescents become aware of their limitations, are critical of themselves and look critically at their own drawings. They are often so critical of the drawings that they finally stop drawing. At this age, adolescents often have a certain preference for or aversion to expressing themselves creatively. Some of them have talent and are praised for this by teachers and fellow students. Criticism and self-criticism are deadly for creative development.

The computer and its possibilities for graphic design opened new possibilities of expression, especially for the young. Some parents or teachers reject creative expression by means of a computer because there is no real contact with the material. If adolescents no longer want to draw on paper, the computer gives them new ways of expressing their creativity in colour and form. In addition, adolescents can use these drawings, perhaps with the accompanying text or sounds, to communicate on a global scale. Of course, it would be unhealthy if this were the only form of communication, since it goes without saying that a personal handshake always makes more of an impression than does a name in an e-mail.

It is to be applauded if young people have the opportunity to express their feelings creatively. Stimulating sports and games, music and creative arts both at school and in the adolescent's leisure time can contribute to this. As parents and care providers, we can pick up signals in this creative expression (or lack thereof) about how the adolescent manifests himself in this transitional phase and where any possible conflicts or points of stagnation may lie. We can help adolescents by offering specific means of creative expression. And by giving adolescents the freedom to find their own way while continuing to provide some protection and supervision so that they do not have the feeling that they are alone.

Case illustration

The parents of a fourteen-year-old boy asked if I could help their son. There were a lot of problems at school because he was aggressive and prone to fighting, and his classmates kept away from him. If things continued this way, he would be expelled from school. When this young man came to me, he of course did not at all feel like 'playing'. I completely agreed with him and suggested that we play a game of billiards on the mini-billiards table in my office. I noticed that he wanted to score points and that he literally hit himself in the head whenever he made a mistake. He was keen on winning. He thought I didn't play too badly and he began to thaw a little. In the meantime, we chatted about school and the home situation and I told him about my practice for children and adults. 'Do adults also play?' he asked. 'Yes,' I said, 'they play soccer, they make music, they paint, run, sing and act. And what we're doing now is also playing, isn't it?' 'I think it's childish and besides, there's nothing wrong with me. I am who I am and others have to accept this.'

He continued to come, albeit reluctantly, and we usually played billiards. He didn't even look at the rest of my office. After a few sessions, he told me that he really wanted to go away, to go off into the wide world, to 'beautiful women on a tropical island'. I asked him what that looked like and if he could draw it. 'I can't draw that,' he said. But he could 'draw' a scene in the sandtray with miniature figures, sand and water. There are two beautiful women staring out to sea. A submarine and a pirates' boat with Captain Hook are ready to set sail. A sailor is keeping the watch. There are dangerous sharks in the water. The voyage to adulthood can begin!

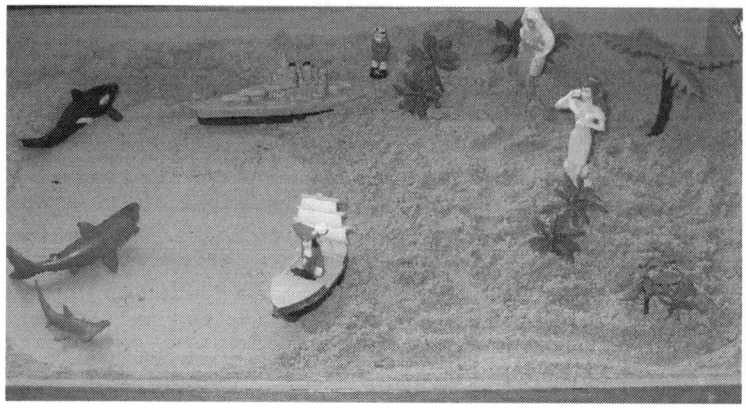

CHAPTER 9

COLOURS, FORMS AND LAYOUT

In the previous chapters, we used developmental psychology to examine the more noticeable characteristics of drawings made by children in various phases of childhood and adolescence. In this chapter, we will discuss more general characteristics, such as colour, form and layouts. We will see that colours, forms and the place of an object on the paper all have symbolic significance and that we can find the source of this significance. Some knowledge of the origins of the significance of these symbols can aid us when we look at children's drawings and want to know more about what they have to tell us.

9.1 The symbolic significance of colours

Parents often notice that their children have a preference for a certain colour. They then wonder, for example, 'If my child uses a lot of black, does that mean her or she is depressed?' The answer to this question can be found below in the discussion about the colour black. Most children use colours in their drawings; in the earliest drawings, they seem to choose colours at random and without preference, but they gradually show a preference for the primary colours such as red, yellow and blue.

As we noted earlier in the discussion of coloured areas, by the age of three, children begin to use all of the colours. After this, they consciously choose a certain colour. It is important to give children not only the primary colours but also black and white when they are drawing or painting. The primary colours can be mixed to make all other colours. Up to the age of four or five, form and colour are more important that content; in fact, a meaning is often given only after the drawing has been finished.

The colourful drawings of a four-year-old resemble modern art by, for example, Karel Appel, because the symbolic emotional value is prominent. Just as the child experiences the world around him as formless and depicts it as such in his drawings, the artist is able to capture the formlessness of the modern world in his art. The child uses his natural instincts; the artist uses his inner sources of inspiration.

The use of colours in children's drawings certainly has a special significance, and below we will discuss the symbolic significance of various colours. It should be said in advance that there is not just one explanation for each colour. As was extensively discussed at the beginning of this book, it is in the nature of symbols to have opposite meanings, just as in the natural conditions of life there is shadow only when the sun shines. Contradictions are found in nature and in people, as we can see, for example, in a love-hate relationship.

Our senses know that something is warm only when we have experienced cold. We are aware that we live because we know that we will die. The symbolic meaning of a colour always has a certain dynamics, a movement between one point and another. Opposites are not value judgments but rather they are opposite activities. The symbolic significance of a colour was not thought of by man, but, just like mythological stories, music, dance and artistic expression, it is naturally anchored in man. We cannot invent colour symbols; we can search for a suitable symbolic colour. Both universal and personal circumstances play a role in the emotional value of a colour symbol. For example, a child suffering from leukaemia may avoid the colour red (Susan Bach '*Life paints its Own Span*'). Or a child that has just been given a new red sweater may draw himself in red that day.

9.2 Psychological investigations into colour

Much psychological research has been done on the significance of colour. The influence of colours on humans has become increasingly recognized, and there are many psychological reasons for using colours in today's advertising, fashion, traffic and politics. Colours have a physiological effect on the body because electromagnetic energy and vibrations differ per colour. Colours are formed in our eyes but light rays are felt by our bodies. An experiment has shown that even a blind person can sense (evidently by experiencing light rays) the difference in colours in Barnett Newman's large and colourful painting *Who's Afraid of Red, Yellow and Blue*.

Johannes Itten did extensive research on the effects of colours in art, psychology and physiology (*The Elements of Color* 1970). He wrote, *'Color is life: for a world without colors appears to us as dead. Colors are primordial ideas, children of the aboriginal colorless light and its counterpart, colorless darkness. As flames beget light, so light engenders color. Colors are the children of light, and light is their mother. Light, that first phenomenon of the world, reveals to us the spirit and living soul of the world through colors.'*

In 1990 Eva Heller published her research into the symbolic influence of colours in which she combined psychological, symbolic, traditional and cultural points of view. In her book *Farben*, Ingrid Riedel describes the psychological significance of colours in images in art, religion and psychotherapy. She concludes that behind a personal preference or emotional tie to a certain colour there is an archetype with which the person in question then has a connection.

Colours were not invented; they have always existed. Man was introduced to colours in nature: the colour of trees, grass, the sky, water, animals, etc. The human body also has colours: the red of blood, exertion or blushing, the white of cold skin, the yellow of death, the brown of faeces, etc. Colours give rise to related emotions that have always been present naturally. In addition, there are contradictions in each colour. The colour green, for example, can signify growth, vegetation, freshness and health, but there are other shades of green that we associate with the taste of something bitter, tart and poisonous. But here again, we cannot assign absolute positive or negative value judgments. For example, the bilious green of a snake's saliva means that a person can be poisoned, but the colour also warns people that something is poisonous.

When looking at colours in drawings, we must be aware of the significance of the colours as well as what and who is expressed in a certain colour. Do the colours coincide with reality or are there noticeable differences? Does such a difference have a symbolic significance or did the child not have access to all of the colours (paint, pencils or felt markers)? Until about the age of six, children may colour an object any colour, depending on their imagination and the coloured pencil nearest to them. At the same time, most children can consciously choose for a certain colour. It also depends on whether a child has an interest in colouring and drawing. What is certain is that, from the age of four, children may have a preference for a certain colour with the symbolic significance attributed to it. We can also see a child's preference for a colour in his or her choice of toys and clothes.

Red
The principal significance of the colour red is its ties with life and death. Red can be found in the body and in nature, both of which have always had both a life-giving and a life-threatening significance. Red is connected to *life* because it is the colour of the blood of menstruation (the colour that is absent during pregnancy) and of birth. Red is connected to *death* because, when blood flows out of the body, death follows. Red thus also means *danger*. Red is also the colour of *fire*, an element that gives warmth and enables man to survive the cold and to cook his raw meat but that can also *destroy*. Here again, life and death are combined. In the Bible, the Apostles speak with tongues of fire, meaning that they were *enthusiastic* and passionate. The red rose, still *a symbol of love*, was an attribute of Venus, the goddess of love. A red traffic sign, such as a stop sign, means something is *dangerous* or *prohibited*, but red can also signify *help* as, for example, in the colour of a fire engine or the Red Cross. In politics, red symbolizes *revolution*, revolt and change. In mythology, Mars, the god of *war*, is a red god.

If children use the colour red, it may be a sign of liveliness, warmth and enthusiasm, but it can also indicate danger, rebelliousness or a cry for help. We have to remain aware that, although we have observed that the child uses the colour red, we can know what *this* colour means for *this* child at *this* moment only when we take into account the child's circumstances and his or her age. The colour red may mean that a child needs help, but it may also mean that a child is able to give help!

Blue
Blue is the colour of the *sky* and of *water*. *Night* is also sometimes experienced as blue, the night in which all colours disappear and everything is invisible. Blue appears in the body that is *cold* or ill. In English the expression 'the blues' refers to a feeling of being *alone* and *unloved*. Blue contains a *free-floating* feeling because it is the colour of the sky and water. Blue in *impersonal* uniforms, such as those worn by the police, civil servants and most men, is business-like and without

imagination. Career-minded people prefer to wear a blue suit; security guards and parking attendants wear a blue *uniform*. The significance of all that blue is that the clothing has *no personal* characteristics. In politics, blue is the colour of reserve and conservatism. On the other hand, dark blue velvet is chic, *erotic* and festive, especially because it sets off gold and silver so well, just as the night sky sets off the stars. Blue is a *heavenly* and thus *divine* colour. In the tombs of Egyptian kings, the graves were often painted blue to indicate the presence of the gods. There were blue gods and goddesses of *love* and dance (Krishna) and gods of wisdom and power (Buddhism). Evil gods in Tibet can appear in *indigo blue*, which is associated with *obsession*, fear and pain.

In children's drawings, sky blue usually appears in the colour of the clouds. A dark cloud is usually a rain cloud. Water is usually light blue. Small children often draw with watery colours, as if they are still swimming in their emotions. Human figures who are coloured blue can have all of the meanings discussed above. We have to look carefully at the colour blue, at what has been coloured (clothes, nature or figures) and at the child's personal circumstances (age, culture, home situation).

Yellow
Yellow is called an *ambivalent* colour with strongly opposing emotions. This is because there is a *warm* yellow such as that of ripened grain, sunflowers, yellow fruits and sand, but also a *sour* yellow such as that of lemons with their sour taste. Someone may actually appear to be yellow because of icterus, a disease of the liver, or they may be yellow in the figurative sense of being cowardly. Yellow sulphurous clouds are *threatening* to our health and a yellow sky can be seen when a thunderstorm threatens. In *spring*, we see the yellow of daffodils and primroses. And at Easter, yellow is the colour of *resurrection* from the dead. We know the warm colour yellow from the colour of sweet honey, the sun and *gold*. Van Gogh used the colour yellow to express the warmth of the sun. In mythology, yellow gods were the gods of *light* and spring. Helios, the sun god, had a shiny yellow robe. The Aztec's corn god was a sun god who embodied *fertility*, dance and pleasure. In painting, we can find an aureole of *holiness* in the colour yellow. Christ was depicted as the Light of the World and framed in a wreath of light. The yellow colour of gold was a symbol of *perfection, revelation and immortality*. Buddhist monks dressed in yellow to show their renunciation

of material things and their devotion to the spiritual as well as their association with *wisdom* and insight.

A child who uses yellow in his or her drawings expresses liveliness and warmth. Children almost always colour the sun yellow (sometimes with a bit of orange). An excessive use of yellow in drawings may indicate a great deal of energy (too warm) or hyperactivity. A certain bright yellow indicates anger (poisonous) or jealousy (sour).

Black
Although black is not a real colour but rather the result of the absorption of colours, we will describe black as experienced in nature and by mankind. Black is experienced in the *night* and in *darkness*. In nature, we see that everything is *blackened* after a fire. There are black fruits such as raspberries and blackberries. Animals that are black, such as the black panther, the raven and the black cat, are often considered negative, *dangerous* or omens of danger. Black clothing is often a sign of *power*, such as the uniform worn by the Nazi SS to emphasize their power. Today, black is often worn by *tough* men (and women) and by sexual sadists. Black is also a sign of *mourning*, sadness and depression. Adolescents often wear black clothes as a sign of being tough and *rebellious*. If we remember that the colour black actually contains all colours, we can understand that black also has many coloured emotions (see also the black and white drawings by adolescents). Black is the colour of the *earth*, the dark hole to which the *dead* return but where *new life* can blossom, just as a seed in the dark earth develops and matures. Black is the *opposite* of white. We still see opposites in black and white in the clothes of the bride and groom and in the ying-yang principle.

There may be many reasons why a child uses a lot of black in a drawing. The child may be depressed or sad and may hide colours (emotions) in black. However, black is commonly used by toddlers and pre-school children in a phase of rebellion, tough behaviour and a struggle for power, something that may be difficult for parents but is necessary for the child. If we understand why something is black in relation to the child's behaviour, we can react adequately. And we should not divide things into one emotion or another since both emotions (such as depressed and rebellious) may be present simultaneously.

White

Like black, white is not really a colour; it is the opposite of black. White is experienced in nature as the *light* of the sun, the moon and the stars. Because we cannot look directly into the light of the sun, the sun was regarded as *divine* light. White appears in nature as snow, milk, eggs and salt. White is the colour of the *end* into which all colours disappear. The white colour of the *corpse* and the *ghostly* white that exists between nothing and something. White is emptiness, nothing. If life is colourless, it is meaningless, sad and empty. But white is also *fresh* and *new*, as is the bride's virginal white. The white of snow where no one has walked is visibly beautiful and *virginal*. An empty sheet of paper is also white. A white egg signifies *fertility* and white salt *wisdom* and *cleansing*.

If a child paints with white he may be expressing emptiness or stagnation. A sheet of paper that is empty or partially empty may indicate a feeling or an aspect that is as yet unknown, unconscious or unripe.

Mixed colours

The three basic colours red, blue and yellow can be mixed to form new colours.

Green

The colour green is made by mixing *blue* and *yellow*. Because the significance of blue (distance and coolness) is mixed with the significance of yellow (warmth and light), both of these significances are *neutralized* in the new colour green.

Green is the colour of *hope*. *New green* in the fields gives the hope of the next harvest. Green grass invites us to lie down, *rest* or dream. The green of trees reminds us of *growth*, development and the fruits that trees can bear. There is the green woods where the sun shines through the leaves and the *dark*, unknown woods in which we can get lost. Among peoples where green was rare, such as among desert tribes, green meant trees, water, an oasis. Water enabled them to survive in the desert. In tropical and primeval forests, the forests were experienced differently because vegetation here overgrew the space where people could live. *Green nature* was both giving and nourishing as well as *devouring*. The element of water plays an important role in nature's becoming green. The green environment that has become increasingly important for our survival is seen as *clean* and *healthy*. Political parties focusing on environmental issues almost always use the word 'green' in their parties' names. In advertising, green is used for healthy products. Green often means a *new beginning*. In many stories of creation, the world begins with the creation of nature, trees and bushes. In today's jargon, someone who is 'green' is an *inexperienced* beginner. The green Tara (Tibet) is the goddess of *rest* and *relaxation*. The Aztecs attributed immortality to a green stone; this stone was placed in the mouth of a corpse as a sign of the *renewing power* of the green life.

In the Middle Ages, Hildegard von Bingen wrote about the healing effects of the colour green, especially green grass. In her book *Hildegard von Bingen*, Ingrid Riedel cites the following: *'Wisdom is the natural order of creation. It is made concrete in the weight of the wind, the measure of water, the law of rain, the path of the clouds'*. The mediaeval verses and songs written by Hildegard are very popular again today. Hildegard wrote about the green goddess (Sophie) and the order of nature that was a sign of divine creation.

Children give vegetation, such as grass and trees, the natural colour green. The use of green in drawings usually has a positive, healthy significance because it expresses growth and vitality. On the contrary, soft green points to a certain tenderness and virginity. There is a sort of hesitant beginning. Dark green points to something that can overpower. Bilious green is a signal of danger and illness (turning green with envy). Such a colour may appear in a secretive place in a drawing, a bit unexpected but certainly noticeable!

Purple
This colour, made from *blue* and *red*, carries both heat and cold, which leads to a sort of *tension*. The significance of red and blue is suppressed by purple and often means a form of emotional suppression. The colour of mourning and *sadness* is often expressed in purple. And figures who call forth feelings of tension or ambivalence, such as magicians or wizards, often wear purple. Purple is frequently seen in children's drawings as an expression of passivity and sadness.

Orange
Orange is made by mixing yellow and red. It is the colour of the rising and setting sun, a beautiful orange glow that exudes warmth and feeling. It is also the colour of the flames of a fire. Orange is a noticeable colour

and can be seen from a distance. The sun in children's drawings is often both orange and yellow. Orange represents warmth, optimism and hope. But it can also be an invasive colour. In the Netherlands, 'royal orange' refers to the House of Orange from which the Dutch monarchy is descended.

Brown

Brown is a combination of red, yellow and blue. In nature, it is the colour of earth and faeces and of the autumn. Brown is an earth colour and is associated with Mother Earth. The colour brown, combining the significance of red (blood and danger), yellow (light and warmth) and blue (distance and coolness), produces a mixture of feelings that can contradict one another. Children who use a lot of brown in their drawings often have hidden, contradictory feelings. A preference for brown may indicate a deep relationship with Mother Earth or a need for warmth and security. Brown is also the colour of faeces, and a brown drawing can also indicate ongoing potty training (see also the drawing in chapter 4 in which messing about with paint is discussed).

9.3 Colours and alchemy

Jungian analytic theory assigns a deeper psychological significance to certain colours that derives from the study of alchemy. The chemical process of transforming stone into gold (as a metaphor for an inner process of the psyche) is the transformation by heating primordial existence (the stone as primordial material) into divine philosophical wisdom (gold). During the transformation, four elements (earth, air, fire and water) and three colours (black, white and red) are present. The first phase of darkness and chaos is black (*nigredo*) into which all colours have been absorbed. Under the influence of the glow of fire (rood=*rubedo*), the material turns white (*albedo*) in which all of the colours are again present so that gold, divine wisdom, can be created.

A description of the complicated philosophy and theories of alchemy goes beyond the scope of this book. Nevertheless, the old and wise symbols of alchemy can be meaningful for a deeper understanding of the significance of colours in children's drawings if, for example, we see that a child is in a period of 'blackness'. We can then imagine that black is needed to initiate a period of transformation. And that a safe and firm (alchemist's) oven is needed in which the 'fire' can burn brightly. We have to be confident that the (cooking) process will follow its own logical course so that we do not open this oven too early (exposing it to the outside world) and cause an explosion. We have to safeguard the flame so that it does not die out or become too hot. When everything has 'burned itself out' and all of the colours are to be found in the white ash, a transformation in the material (the personality) can occur.

Case illustration

A ten-year-old girl came to therapy with vague physical complaints such as stomach aches, headaches and concentration problems. Her mother had died when the girl was a year and a half. Her father cared for her for a few years and then she went to various foster homes. She had difficulty making contact and often felt alone. After months of therapy in which a relationship of trust was established and feelings of isolation were expressed, there followed a period in which she used black paint, black felt markers and black pencils to make formless and boundless drawings. She also made patterns with black and white dominoes in the sandtray. At that point, I felt that her use of black was therapeutically necessary. Her feeling of loss could finally be expressed. And then she discovered red and made a sort of campfire from red clay and red crepe paper. I was amazed and delighted when she put a 'gold ball' into the fire, a round gold candle that stayed lit for the rest of the session. After this period, more natural drawings and subjects were depicted, such as trees and animals. And the inner contact with the archetypal inner mother was re-established in the form of caring for baby dolls in the doll house.

For clarity's sake, it should be said again that in Jungian analytical therapy that reaches to the deeper layers of the psyche, it is strictly necessary that a child – in the therapeutic situation – is free to choose what he or she wants to do and how he or she wants to do it. That means that no assignments can be given and no suggestions to do or make something can be made. The adult (therapist or care provider) may think that the time has come for the child to make or draw something in a certain way, but he or she will not make any suggestions, proposals or even hints. We must trust that the child is able to find a solution that we may not have seen. It is always surprising to observe how creative a child is (and this is also true of adults who go through a similar creative process). Each of us has the ability to find creative solutions for problems that we encounter. This part of the world of the psyche is called the 'inner child' in Jungian terms.

When a child has to learn something at school, such as drawing in perspective or copying figures or landscapes, superficial functions of the psyche and the intellect are called into play and the deeper layers of the psyche are not reached.

9.4   The symbolic meaning of the basic forms

The basic forms as we know them in drawings also derive from nature, the cosmos and the human body. The spiral, the circle and the cross are discovered by the child in their first drawings; their significance has already been described in chapter 3. The significance of these forms remains but becomes more subtle as the child grows older. The square and the triangle are the last of the basic forms drawn by a child. This is in keeping with the constructive, intellectual and physical skills needed to draw these forms and – as with the earlier discoveries of spirals, crosses and circles – with the psychological significance of the square and the triangle.

In several of his works, Jung gave a psychological and archetypal explanation of the significance of the basic forms (Jung 1966, 1987, 1991). Another detailed explanation is given in Ingrid Riedel book *Forms* (1985). And Ursula Eschenbach (Hrsg) also researched and explained the significance of various basic forms in her book *Das Symbol im therapeutisch Prozesz bei Kinder und Jugendlichen* (1978).

1. The square

Like the triangle, the square has to be constructed, something that requires a certain amount of intelligence. In the material world, the square expresses the *perimeters* of *possession*. From the moment that man began to develop as an individual, material possessions were marked off with a line, a fence or a border. A demarcation in its negative sense can be a jail. A child not only draws a square, but he or she can also play with or in a square. The important characteristic of the mathematical demarcations of a square is that limits are determined. In a certain period, children play games with borders in the school playground or in their neighbourhood. Somewhere a line is drawn and the other side is not allowed to cross that line. Or the rules say that you can or cannot walk on a certain line. In such games, children learn to respect the limits of the other, to protect their own borders or to trespass on those of others.

Another characteristic of the square is its *four sides*. By walking in a square, the child experiences the four different directions and symbolically learns (first with the body and then with the psyche) that you can consider something from various sides once you adopt a different point of view.

The *cube* is derived from the square and has more dynamism and fascination. The cube is an unfathomable form that is known as a dice having both visible and invisible sides. The dice can roll, move and come to a stop. Once the dice has stopped moving, one's fate is sealed because 'the die has been cast'. When playing a game with dice, the child practices the whims of fate and learns that something is a certain amount, no more and no less. A child can accept this from about the age of three or four.

Another special form containing a square is the *labyrinth*, which uses its rectilinearity in an attempt to dynamically open the narrow limitations of the square (Riedel, *Forms*, p. 23). The labyrinth is known in many cultures as a form of meditation in which a solution is found for questions or problems. In a *maze*, children (and adults) can experience the excitement of looking for an exit and the relief when the exit has been found, which is why the maze is still so popular in playgrounds or at the fair.

Many computer games are also based on the need to find a solution. However, the paths and the goal are sometimes commercially constructed with the purpose of keeping the child in the game without their being able to reach the goal. Parents should realize that, although computer games can be good, they should not contain such intentional constructions since some children can become so fascinated by the inaccessibility of the goal that they enjoy few of the positive experiences involved in finding a solution.

A child who draws a square around a house or himself marks off his possession or himself from the outside world. It is sometimes good to establish boundaries and, at other times, good to open these boundaries. Drawing a square means that a child is able to make and respect boundaries. Drawing a labyrinth points to a child's search for a solution and also helps the child to concentrate when trying to achieve his or her goal.

2. The triangle

The triangle is a dynamic man-made form that appears in nature only in crystal. In many cultures, triangles are symbols of *male* and *female*. In old religions (Hinduism) the triangle is drawn with its apex at the bottom for the female and its apex at the top for the male. The triangle's connection with male and female is also known among the Zulus. Here, the apex at the top signifies an unmarried male and an apex at the bottom an unmarried woman. Men and women wear triangular bead necklaces, and the colours also signify whether or not they are eligible or if they are in love with a certain person (Stan Schoeman '*Eloquent beads, the semantic of a Zulu art form*'). In our culture, children and adults wear a triangle as jewellery, although the extent to which such jewellery unconsciously signifies the old meaning goes beyond the scope of this book.

A triangle with a special significance is the Star of David, a symbol consisting of two entwined and superimposed triangles that had to be worn by the Jews as a stigma during World War Two. Today in the Western world, the triangle as a symbol of male and female is not very common other than the pink triangle used as a sign of liberation by Gay Pride, a sign deriving from the pink triangle worn by homosexuals imprisoned in Nazi concentration camps.

A more familiar triangle is the one with its apex at the top that is used to show that something is *forbidden* or *dangerous*, such as in traffic signs or on bottles containing dangerous fluids. The *number three* is used to indicate a time span such as past-present-future or birth-life-death. The number three stands for action. In fairy tales, the number three can be found in the number of trials that a person must go through or the number of riddles that have to be solved.

In children's drawings, the first clearly constructed triangle is the *roof of a house*, something that also expresses the triangular relationship between father-mother-child. Adolescents sometimes construct drawings with triangles, which often means that the adolescent is looking for a new relationship with his or her parents. Drawing triangles as decoration or abstractions may indicate tension in relationships with others.

Case illustration
During one of my courses on the significance of children's drawings, a participant brought a drawing done by her fourteen-year-old daughter. It was a drawing of constructed triangles, all of which had been given a different colour. The mother told me that her daughter had been making drawings like this one for weeks and she asked me what the significance might be. I asked her if there were any problems in the triangular relationship father-mother-child. That was, in fact, the case. The parents were considering a divorce but had not yet made a decision. In these drawings, the daughter showed that she too was involved in these problems even though she had not yet spoken about them.

9.5   The symbolic significance of the layout

In the beginning, children draw randomly on a piece of paper without choosing the top, the bottom, right or left. Subjects and objects are given names even though the figures do not have to resemble them. After the age of four, children consciously begin to draw more in keeping with reality and objects are given a somewhat fixed or correct place on the paper. A house, a tree, animals and people are drawn in the middle, to the left or to the right. The sun appears at the top in the sky and flowers are drawn at the bottom in the earth. This reflects the child having more control over himself and the world around him.

Children can also have their drawings narrate a story, as was discussed earlier in the section on drawings by children between the ages of seven and ten. They can draw events taken from daily life, such as a school trip, their holiday, what they want to be when they grown up, etc. Such drawings have little perspective; objects seem to be placed at random. This is similar to the previously discussed paintings from the Middle Ages that depicted stories of religious events, the life of a famous person, etc. Although the place of an object on the paper seems to be a random one, this same randomness gives it a symbolic significance.

The symbolic significance of the layout was not thought of by humans but, as with all of the previously mentioned symbols, it is anchored in nature and in man. It is only natural to draw earthly things at the bottom of the paper (we stand with our feet on the ground) and the sun and stars at the top. We look down when we are embarrassed (earth, dark) and we lift our heads when we speak to God (exalted, light). Much psychological research has been done on the layout of two-dimensional forms. Spatial schemes based partially on a study of art history have been named for Grünwald, Susan Bach, and Rudolf Mitch and have been further developed by Ingrid Riedel (*'Bilder'* p. 31).

The most well-known symbolic significance of a surface is that the right side concerns the future and the left side the past. Tests for this left/right symbolism established that most (right-handed) people, when asked to draw a line for the future, drew a diagonal line going from left up to right and that, when asked to draw a line for the past, they drew a diagonal line from right down to left (Riedel). However, this did not give unambiguous results for left-handed people since some of these drew in the opposite direction and others did not. But this shows that we should not be too eager to take a definitive point of view without considering all of the possibilities present in humans.

These same significances of layout can also be found in studies of religious drawings and iconography. In these studies, a symbolic significance is attributed to an area. The paper (or canvas) is divided into four zones. The top, bottom, left, right and the four corners with their diagonals have symbolic significances that derive from a certain source and that are the same in these studies. These divisions are not completely valid for a three-dimensional figure. There are similarities but, in figures in space, above and below, for example, do not have to be expressed on a flat surface but can also be higher or lower or on top of or underneath. The divisions found in these studies have been made especially for a flat surface in an enclosed space. When using these interpretations of layouts, it is important not to think in rigid divisions. Gestalt's axiom that 'the whole is more than the sum of the parts' certainly applies here as a warning not to become entangled in details. As in music, we can hear a melody only when the various notes are played in harmony with one another. We can find this harmony only when we have considered all of the possibilities and have found the last pieces of the puzzle. Keeping this in mind, we can take a brief look at the significances of schematic layouts as described in literature and use them to understand the significance of a drawing.

The zones
Top: The top part of the paper indicates the heavens, divinity, light, fire, the spirit and the psyche.

Bottom: The bottom part indicates the base, rooting, depth, earth and water.

Left side: This is the side of the past, desires, the subconscious, darkness, returning and regression.

Right side: This is the future, consciousness and activity.

The corners
A more detailed division takes into account the four corners. It is assumed that the left top corner belongs to the (archetypal) father and the right bottom corner to the (archetypal) mother. The left bottom corner is the collective unconsciousness and the right top corner the development of consciousness and a conscience.

Directions
We can also look at the direction in which people and things in a drawing are moving since this can indicate the direction a development may take. Movement from left to right is towards the future and reality; movement from right to left is towards the past and the subconscious. Young children usually draw people and cars moving from right to left: they focus on their feelings and the subconscious. After about the age of seven, people and cars more often move from left to right: they move towards the present and reality. According to the symbolic significance of layouts, this is the result of the fact that, for the most part, small children still find themselves on the left side, the side of the subconscious and the past. As the intellect grows, children begin to focus on the future and the reality and activities of the external world as represented by the right side of the paper. In general, children draw from the bottom of the page up; as they increase in age, the bottom of a drawing is placed higher, meaning that the child's perspective has risen and his or her view has expanded.

The middle
As already described in the discussion on the circle and its core (chapter 3), finding a middle point is an important psychological process. As Jung writes in *Man and his Symbols*: 'Among the mythological representations of the Self one finds much emphasis on the four corner of the world, and in many pictures the Great Man is represented in the center of a circle divided into four.' (Von Franz: p.230)(p. 175).

The middle point of a square surface is the beginning of a mandala form because the mandala (which means 'magic circle') is made by emphasizing the four corners with a special significance. The special significance of such a middle point is known in various religions (Tibetan, Christian) and mythological stories of creation as well as in the architecture of churches, cathedrals and other buildings. And even in modern drawings or buildings (such as a soccer stadium), we look for the middle point because this is the safest.

If a drawing has a certain balance because of the use of the corners, this indicates that there is a tendency to find a middle point. In Jungian theory, this middle point signifies the previously mentioned Self. The symbolic significance of a figure, colour or form exactly in the middle of the drawing is an extremely personal one for the individual who made the drawing.

9.6 Learning to look at the layouts of a drawing

We can look at a child's drawing by ourselves, with others or with the child. A narrative drawing can be made as an assignment (make a drawing about your holiday) or spontaneously. We may ask what is going on in the drawing, but we should never answer this question ourselves without first knowing something about the circumstances surrounding the child. We do not know if the child made an exciting drawing because of something he or she read in the paper or a book, or if they heard a story from someone else, or if they experienced the situation themselves. If a child draws an exciting story because of something he or she has heard, we can conclude that the story made quite an impression on the child. Drawing about it can lessen the fear. An exciting story compensates for one's own fears, which is why children (and adults) read exciting books and obituaries and why people go to witness disasters and accidents. The underlying psychological thought is 'thankfully, it didn't happen to me'. We can also see an exciting drawing as a sign that the child is drawing something he or she is afraid of, such as an accident or aggression.

If we look again at the narrative drawing in chapter 7 (p.115), we can examine it with the knowledge of the symbolic significance of colours, forms and layouts discussed above.

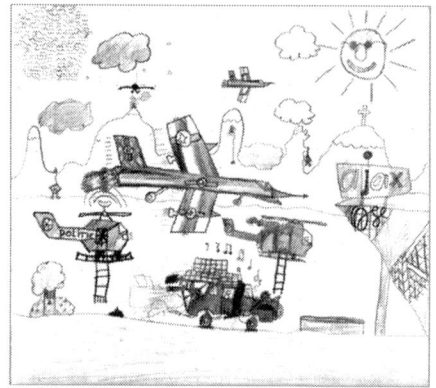

We see that all four corners have been filled. There is a flock of birds at the top left; at the top right, the sun with its sunglasses and teeth is shining above a mountain with a cross; at the bottom left, a special tree with roots and a crown that almost reflect each other and a police helicopter; at the bottom right, the triangular roof of the Ajax soccer stadium; in the middle, a car with music coming from it. The planes in the drawing are mostly red, the clouds are blue and the sun is yellow.

Significance

This drawing has a great amount of symbolic significance, much of which is by now already familiar to the reader: birds, planes, clouds, sun, tree, car, triangle, a cross and mountains. The mountains are steep and covered with snow, which means that the will to achieve is strong and (emotional) life perhaps cold. The symbolism of stone is in keeping with that of a mountain (hard, steep and difficult to climb). The form of the mountains is both male (phallic) and female (breasts). There is a cross on the mountain at the right. Perhaps a sign that the top has been reached? But a cross can also be a sign of death. The rays of the sun show that the child has freed himself of his ties to the mother and that the father's characteristics (action, conscience, consciousness) are present. A special tree at the bottom left is not well-rooted and the trunk is perhaps not strong enough to bear the weight of the tree. There is also a hollow in the tree. The child may have tried to draw the shadow of the tree on the ground and perhaps there are apples on the ground. Nevertheless, the shape of the tree is strange, and we may wonder if something strange happened at the beginning of the child's life (in the unconscious phase of his existence).

We also see that there is an explosive force of a plane (and of the child himself) in the middle of the drawing that moves from left to right and that is thus oriented towards the future. Looking at the left side of the drawing, the side of the past (or the subconscious), we see that help was needed and that there was sadness, danger or illness. We can also see this in the figures on the mountains who are standing or hanging in dangerous spots and in the helicopter with its rope ladder and stretcher. The future or reality (right side) looks sunnier, has more energy, perhaps more aggression, it offers a challenge in the world of sports (Ajax) and perhaps the bleachers with spectators in the stadium can both watch and watch over the child (in the corner of the archetypal mother).

The space on the paper has been used well except for the bottom edge where a light green stripe has been coloured. That might mean that the things that are closest, such as (mother) earth and water (the source of life and feelings) are empty or unripe, and this might be connected to the unhappy left side. At the moment of drawing, the child made the story of the drawing from a higher (and newer) perspective on life.

A well-filled piece of paper may indicate vitality and a strong interaction with the surrounding world, but it may also indicate a strong desire for a fuller life. Consequently, the child creates this for himself. The significance of this drawing with a story is not complete because the real circumstances surrounding the child could not be given here. It is just an example of how we can look at the form and content of a drawing, but we must again stress that there is always an invisible aspect in the symbolic interpretation of a drawing: that which is not yet known or of which we are unconscious or have no words to express. This is true of both the person who made the drawing and the person interpreting the drawing.

CHAPTER 10

ANIMALS AND FANTASY FIGURES

10.1 The animalistic phase

At about the age of three or four, the age at which children first begin to draw tadpoles, they also begin to draw their first animals. In this phase, drawings of humans often resemble those of animals; in fact, there is no visible difference between the two since animals are given human forms and facial expressions.

Together with the vegetative phase, the animalistic phase is the most primitive phase in a child's development (*anima* = animal). Our relationship with animals dates from before birth, when the foetus in the uterus resembled a fish or a bird, and from our evolutionary roots. Instincts 'know' more than does everyday knowledge. Our primordial ancestors learned to survive by using their instincts. They saw and knew what was dangerous and what was beneficial to them. In the animalistic phase, man was (and the child is) strongly connected to instinctive wisdom. This is no longer the phase of expectation and vegetating, but the phase of discovery and activity.

Natural instincts play a role in the animalistic phase. The child is aided by animal instincts, instinctive impulses anchored in man, such as the animal's 'knowing' that it has to build a nest or has to flee in the face of danger. Thousands of years of ancestral experiences of surviving in the natural world have been stored in our body's organs and in our psyche so that man, and especially the young child who is still so close to unconscious nature, has been able to survive. The child who is still in the animalistic phase 'knows' nature and animals with a knowledge that has not been taught to him.

Up until the age of four or five, a child finds himself in the magical and animalistic phase described above. This means that the child experiences animals and nature as having a 'soul'. Children easily make contact with animals. Most stuffed toys are animals. As children age, their knowledge of reality grows so that they can differentiate between fantasy and reality;

nevertheless, magical and animalistic thoughts continue to play a role for quite some time.

10.2   The symbolic significance of animals

In Gmeling's book *Mama ist ein Elephant,* a book about the meaning of children's drawings, it is assumed that the child acquires his or her knowledge of animals from books or other sources such as fairy tales, children's literature and everyday speech (p. 47). However, it seems unlikely that children have gained this knowledge intellectually. Rather, this knowledge comes from the collective unconscious, the experiences of our primordial ancestors, which causes people to react naturally in certain ways.

In these sorts of drawing games (or Draw-Your-Family as an Animal-test) it is often quite tempting to jump to conclusions about personality traits of people in the child's surroundings. However, the symbolic significance of an animal is not unambiguous since every animal has its positive, negative and even dangerous aspects for man. All sorts of traits can be expressed as symbols in an animal, but it is also possible that the child wants to express only one trait when he draws a certain animal. And, as we have already explained in previous chapters, symbolic significance cannot simply be taken from a book about symbols because a number of factors play a role. All of these considerations may suggest that it is impossible to interpret a drawing, but it is possible to take a wide view of the many alternatives. Nevertheless, we must accept the fact that we cannot possibly know or explain everything because the strength of a symbol also lies in its unknown aspects.

The combination man-animal can be traced back to the rituals and artistic expressions of our ancestors. Man created a man-animal combination if a human characteristic was considered so special that it could be compared only to an animal. One of the oldest examples of a human animal or an animalistic human is the sphinx, with its reclining body of a lion and the head of a woman. The Sphinx at the pyramids in Egypt was built about 4500 years ago.

The combination of a lion's body and a woman's head points to the intensely strong power that a woman was assumed to have: namely, the power of a lion.

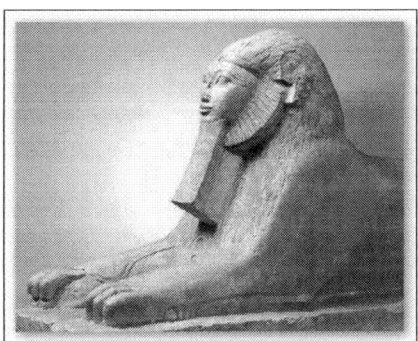
www.touregypt.net/featurestories/sphinx1.htm

There are many more examples of animals in human forms, such as those in the drawings and hieroglyphics in the Egyptian tombs. Animal traits, both positive and negative, were expressed as divine traits. For example, the Egyptian god Sobek, the god of rivers and lakes, was depicted with the head of a crocodile.

In general, the crocodile has a dangerous and devouring significance in mythologies, legends and religions. An example of this is the Egyptian god Ammit, the god who devoured the soul of the deceased if he or she was not admitted to the underworld. In Uganda, crocodiles were used to test a person's guilt or innocence. The accused was brought to a river and forced to cross it; if attacked by crocodiles, he was guilty.

In reality, the crocodile actually is a dangerous and devouring animal. But the mother crocodile is also an animal that for months patiently guards the eggs in her nest and that, once the eggs have hatched, takes the baby crocodiles in her mouth to the water, where she then protects them for another few weeks. Because of this, the crocodile is also regarded in some myths and cultures in Africa and South America as a symbol of fertility and it represents a positive maternal aspect.

A child who draws his or her mother as a crocodile in the 'draw your family as an animal' game may want to express the mother as dangerous and devouring, but it can also be an expression of security and protection by an (overly) concerned mother. It is also possible that the child sometimes experiences the mother as devouring and sometimes as protective. Positive and negative feelings can alternate or exist simultaneously. Animals especially can contain these contradictions, which is why animals played a large role in the emotions of our ancestors and do so again in those of small children.

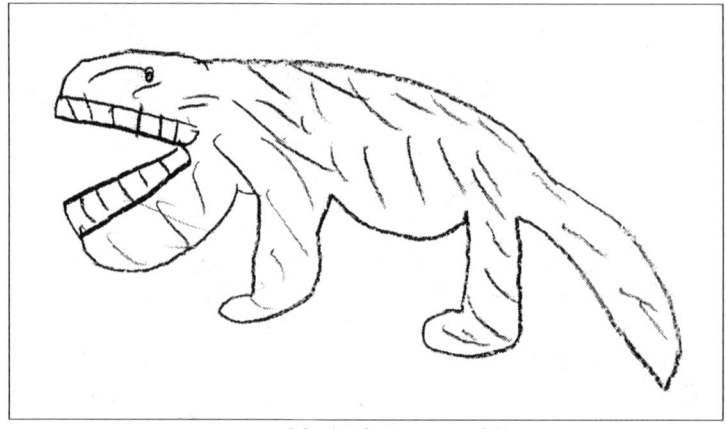

crocodile (girl, 8 years old)

All primitive peoples have rituals in which humans dress as animals to show that they possess these animal traits.

Our ancestors met animals who threatened them, but they also hunted animals in order to survive. Man had a natural relationship with a cow or a goat that gave milk, with chickens and birds that laid eggs and with fish that could be eaten. Animals also shared the home, could be petted and trusted and were playmates for children. There were also animals that helped people with, for example, their tasks in the field or in transporting heavy loads. And, of course, there are stories of animals such as dolphins, whales or turtles that saved human lives.

C.G. Jung called the body a museum of organs that has a long evolutionary history containing millions of years of experiences in living together with animals. Genetics is only now discovering the facts of which Jung, in his theories about the collective unconscious, was convinced. In *The seven daughters of Eve* by Brian Sykes, a genetic scientist at the Institute of Molecular Medicine in Oxford, Sykes wrote, *'Every cell in our body contains genetic material from a woman who lived 70,000 years ago in Italy.'*

Contact with animals was important in the development of our ancestors' instincts. We can now understand why young children have an expressed preference for animals. The animalistic phase, the phase in which a child feels especially attracted to animals, is important for the development of a child's instincts. Animals help the child to come into contact with the instinctive traits of his or her own psyche and, as the child becomes increasingly more conscious of his or her own will, the instincts are integrated into forming the personality. The individual will is of a higher intellectual order in the development towards becoming conscious and can come into existence only when instinctive reactions have been assimilated.

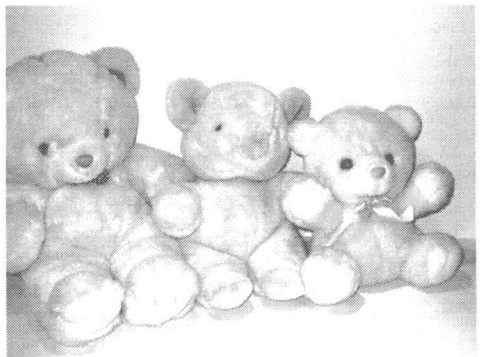

(stuffed teddy bears)

If we want to gain the trust of a small child who is afraid, we often use an animal such as a teddy bear or a live rabbit. A child understands and trusts an animal sooner than he does another human. Those working with difficult children also claim that it is possible to make deeper contact with such children when using an animal as an intermediary. In a recent experiment in the United States, children with reading problems were given a dog that rested against them as they read; the level of their reading achievements increased dramatically (see *Florida Today*, May 2003). We can thus understand why children draw animals with human traits: they can then let animals laugh and talk and they give animals a human appearance.

To understand the deeper psychological significance of an animal in a drawing, we should take into account the instinctive sources from which a child 'knows' how an animal behaves. Of course, a child who has his or her own rabbit, cat or dog has a special experience with and feeling for that animal. Moreover, children often have a natural preference for an animal that answers a certain instinctive need (such as babies who love a sheep that goes 'meh, meh' and strong-willed toddlers love a tiger that goes 'grr, grr'!).

10.3 Stuffed animals as transitional objects

The teddy bear is a popular stuffed animal and the favourite of many children. The teddy bear became a commercial success after the American president Theodore Roosevelt, whose nickname was 'Teddy', admitted that he could not kill a bear during a hunting expedition. In addition, the bear, especially the brown bear, is seen as the primordial mother that protects her young cubs with her life. On the other hand, however, Europeans considered the bear, with its long nails and claws, as a symbol threatening man's well-being. Although there are not many brown bears roaming freely in Europe at the moment, history has shown us that the brown bear was not threatening to humans if it had enough to eat. In North America and Alaska, however, the black bear is still extremely dangerous. This may explain why you do not see many children playing with a black teddy bear. Do children know that the black bear is almost always a dangerous animal that attacks humans without warning? Then it is not just a coincidence that there are hardly any adult-looking black teddy bears for sale, whereas you can buy black baby teddy bears since they are not (yet) dangerous. A brown (or a white) teddy bear is usually a positive maternal symbol and, as a stuffed toy, a sort of substitute for the mother.

D.W. Winnicot studied the significance of a transitional object that the child clutched closely as a remembrance of his or her mother. This object may be a stuffed toy but it can also be something else soft, such as a piece of cloth or a blanket. Intellectually, the child is making the transition from illusions to disillusions; in other words, the child is still in the paradise of the unconscious but is beginning to become conscious of feelings of fear and abandonment.

10.4 Why (stuffed) animals can help

It is a well-known fact in a therapeutic process that children (and adults) who have had a traumatic experience at an early age so that the development of a healthy ego has been impaired may experience a regression in service of the ego (Ernst Kris, *'Psychoanalytic explorations in Art'* 1952). There is a symbolic regression to an earlier phase. In a therapeutic process (such as Sandplay), we can see this when a child reverts to the animalistic phase. The child then plays with toy aquatic animals, such as ducks, fish, snakes and dolphins that are in keeping with the earliest phase of existence in which the child swims in the uterus and where the development of the foetus strongly resembles that of a marine animal. These aquatic animals guide the child to the next phase of development, that of birth and independent breathing and living. In therapy, such a phase may be referred to as 'rebirthing'. Regression does not just happen and it cannot be forced to happen. Expert professional therapeutic knowledge and supervision is needed since the child will otherwise not grow past the animalistic (or other regressive) phase. In short, such a process moves from the primitive earthly instincts (the animalistic stage) via contact with nature, trees and fruit (the vegetative stage) to the relationship with other people (the social and collective stage).

All of these stages can be recognized in a therapeutic (sandplay) process. They are the normal stage of development that a child must pass through for a healthy personality development. We have seen these stages in the development of children's drawings in the previous chapters. If stagnation or something similar happened at a certain stage of a child's development, the child may return to this phase to repeat the experience (for example, in a game or some other form of expression) so that a healthy process of development can ensue. We refer to this as 'regression in service of the ego'.

But animals also play a role in a child's healthy development. If in a certain phase of his or her life a child has an expressed preference for a certain animal (alive or toy), we can better understand the child if we know more about the symbolic significance of that animal. Moreover, we can sometimes more consciously give a child an animal or a toy animal if we know what the symbolic significance of that animal is, which animal traits (instincts) such an animal has and if they meet the needs of the child.

As adults, we often have to discover the natural background of an animal by study and research since, in the course of life, and especially in the last century, it seems as if man has lost his innate knowledge of the natural world. Life in modern cities hardly affords the opportunity to come into contact with animals in their natural habitats, something that impoverishes the natural development of humans. Technology and the exploitation of the environment have put an end to natural conditions; humans and animals can no longer live together, so that there are hardly any remaining examples of the primordial natural world that served as man's example in his development towards consciousness. And because nature is being depleted so quickly and in such a short time, a great many species have already disappeared forever from the planet.

In the previous sections, we have discussed how important animals have been in the development of instincts. If humans no longer have access to the examples of animals, there is the danger that instincts will become unknown and repressed. The force of these animal instincts will be funnelled towards the subconscious, with the danger of their suddenly causing an explosion. Take as an example the dinosaurs that are currently so popular. Since the discovery of the dinosaur's bones and skeletons, humans have begun to fantasize about these animals with which man has never cohabitated. I was told that in the 1980s, Dora Kalff predicted that the dinosaur would somehow make its return because modern man has lost his contact with his primordial instincts. In the 1990s, there were a number of exciting films and stories about the return of the dinosaur. The theme in *Jurassic Park*, in which people are confronted by dinosaurs who had secretly survived, represents man's fear of being faced with old, instinctive, destructive forces. Coming into contact with these dinosaurs (in games, films or drawings) is a symbolic expression of this fear.

It is worthwhile to examine the extent to which, at a certain phase, children who have to deal with old conflicts (perhaps conflicts between the parents or between the parents and the grandparents), the fear of the unknown or the fear of something threatening (such as illness or loss) play with dinosaurs! Experienced (sandplay) therapists say that if children frequently play with or are obsessed by dinosaurs, it often means that the child feels overwhelmed by something large and threatening, that he or she is afraid of certain feelings or that there is a connection to primordial feelings from long ago.

We can recognize the significance of an animal in fairly tales which tell of the hero or heroine being helped by an animal. The deeper significance here is that, in a conflict situation between good and bad, the animal knows which road to take. That means that the decisive factor is our animal instinct. Imagine that there were no longer animals to enable children to recognize their instincts. How would they then learn of the soft, supportive, dangerous, aggressive or beneficial powers that animals represent? If we lose contact with animals, then all animals (all instincts) would continue to live in us as dinosaurs, unknown and terrifying.

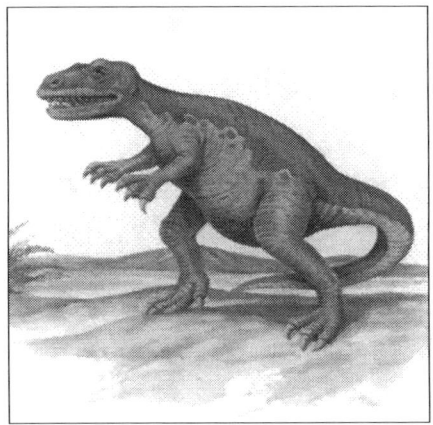

dinosaur

10.5   The significance of fantasy figures

The very colourful fantasy figures that appeal to the imagination and that may appear in children's drawings are often figures known from fairy tales (or popular books or TV series) and that can often be traced back to mythological stories. In chapter 3, we followed the development of children's drawings from non-figurative forms and colours through the drawings of people, animals, trees and the sun up to the more detailed drawings first without and later with perspective.

Children can draw a situation from daily life and from their fantasies and dreams. If we think about our own dreams, then we realize that there are no limits to what can be fantasized. The non-figurative, almost abstract drawings that stem from the pre-verbal period have very little narrative content. From about the age of six, the child's mythological world becomes increasingly overshadowed by reality and the real world around him. The intellect becomes more important, and the universal pre-verbal drawings give way to the more personal interpretations of reality. Children use realistic and self-invented figures and objects to express their fantasies.

In drawings, books and stories, there are fantasy figures that have a strong power of attraction for a certain age group. In the last decade, there have been hundreds of fantasy figures for sale, ranging from comic book figures to figures from Disney films, TV series, and computer and card games. Many of these fantasy figures are popular because they have a deeper symbolic significance that their creators – consciously or unconsciously – made use of (for example, Star Wars or Pokemon). In the past few years, a gigantic toy industry has evolved, one that uses not only fantasy figures but also things taken from reality and duplicated in plastic, stone or ceramics. The predecessor of the world of grown-ups in miniature began with doll houses and tin soldiers, but at the moment almost everything in the world exists in miniature forms, many of which are made in China.

In some forms of therapy, and particularly in Sandplay, these miniatures are used to give the child as wide a range as possible in expressing his or her fantasy world. Sandplay uses not only the realistic world in miniature, such as houses, trees, cars and all sorts of people and animals, but also figures from well-known fairy tales and new modern comic books or TV series. Using these figures and a special sandtray, the child can make a three-dimensional image of his or her fantasy, an image that may be terrifying, chaotic, fragmented, exciting, imaginative, dreamy or realistic and that can depict a fantasy or a realistic scene from the past or the present. The therapist should be able to understand the realistic and the symbolic content of the images and to guide these in a therapeutic process. It should be stated that, without any training in or experience of Sandplay, it is irresponsible to make a collection of miniature figures in a sandtray in the hopes that such a process will occur of itself. Sandplay therapy is a therapy that affects the deep layers of the child's psyche (and of those adults who experience such a process). The influence of this process on the psyche has been well described in D. Kalff's book *Sandplay, a psychotherapeutic approach to the psyche*.

But we do not need to be specialists or therapists to see how and with what a child plays. In a healthy normal environment in which a child plays, whether it be the house or the school, we as parents and teachers can better understand the child if we know more about the background and the significance of a certain fantasy figure. And understanding a child is positive because we feel one with the child. If a child is especially fascinated by a certain game or figure, we can try to discover, together with the child, what this figure represents, which emotions belong to this figure or if there is a connection to myths and fairy tales. We can try to discover this by examining the universal archetypes and the symbolic and personal significance of such a game or figure.

In the sections that follow, we will give examples of fantasy figures that appear again and again in fairy tales, stories, books, TV series and computer games. This is just a selection from the many fantasy figures in the world around us; there are many more of these figures, but these examples show how the symbolic significance of such a figure may be determined. We can try to discover the archetypal figures, the archetypes that are found at all times but with a different appearance or form and that nevertheless have the same contents and significance.

When searching for the symbolic significance of these fantasy figures, we always encounter contradictory meanings. But contradictions are not always only positive or negative. This is because the boundaries of a symbolic significance are not so fixed; they interweave with each other, just like the black and white symbol of ying-yang (male-female) in which the black area penetrates the white area just as much as the white area penetrates the black.

1. Elves

Elves are fantasy figures that are especially attractive to girls of four and five. Naturally, elves are very sweet but they are not unlike a two-year-old toddler who at a certain moment shows that he or she is not only sweet but is also capable of getting his or her own way by being angry and stubborn.

Elves are sweet and childish, but also too naïve and they always remain tiny. Another representative of an elf is the Barbie doll with her ideal appearance. The Barbie doll can be both the child's ideal ('I want to be the sweetest and the prettiest') and the parents' ideal that the child has to conform to. The child may think 'My dad and mum think that I should be sweet and perfect' but he or she may also think 'I'm not so sweet and perfect, but I'd like to be'.

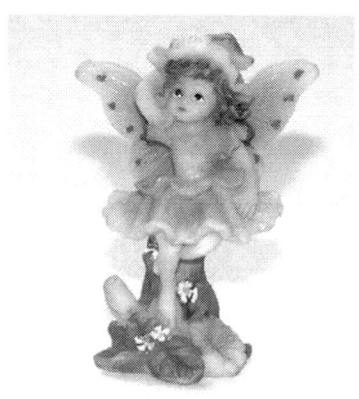

We can determine whether the elf and the Barbie doll play a compensating or a dominating role. A child that always draws elves or one who collects them or wants to be one may become fixated by these elfish traits. At a certain point, we should question whether or not the child has emotionally remained too long in the little (girl and) elf's world. In that case, the child has to be helped and stimulated to grow in his or her development. Being an elf for too long may also be a sign that the child is too naïve or too sweet for his or her age.

2. Fairies

If we see a fairy in a drawing or a game, we usually think of a good fairy, a figure who can help people. But there is also a bad fairy, often forgotten, who can cast an evil spell on people.

Every good fairy in a fairy tale has to contend with a bad fairy, the fairy who is jealous or who was not invited and who therefore had to invite herself. She is the cause of things happening that no one had expected (for example, in *Sleeping Beauty*). The good fairy teaches children that it is good to have wishes and to express them. The bad fairy teaches children that they cannot always depend on getting

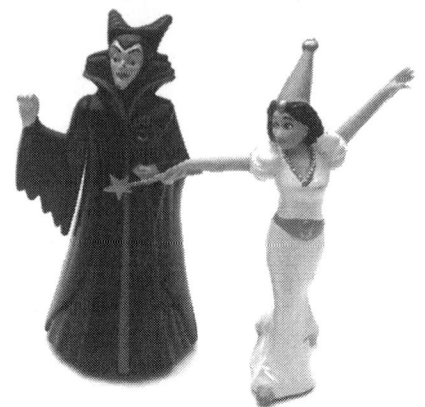

what they wish for. The good and the bad fairy are representatives of the good mother and the bad mother. These are not criteria to evaluate the real, personal mother, but rather they represent the positive and negative feelings that a child has with regard to feelings of protection, nurture, nourishment, etc. The 'bad fairy feelings' help a child to free himself of his parents, accept a loss or become independent.

If a child often plays with fairies, we may wonder what the child's wishes are. Are there circumstances that should be changed? Does the good fairy compensate for things that the child cannot have? It may also be that the child must learn that he cannot always get what he wants. We sometimes see that children who have had a traumatic experience play with the bad fairy. We may think that the child is expressing his feelings of anger, but it also means that the bad fairy is helping the child to accept reality (he did not get what he wanted). The inner negative feeling, that can be so destructive for the child's healthy development, can be projected onto the bad fairy, who has then been given an image. And, as has been shown throughout this book, expressing or giving form to feelings can have a healing effect on the psyche.

3. Witches

The witch is often found in drawings made by both boys and girls. The psychological significance may be found in the realistic situation of a child that has just had an argument with his or her mother and wants to depict her as an old witch.

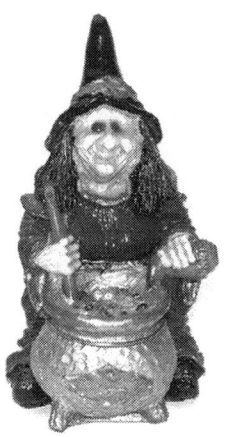

At some point every child experiences the archetypal Negative Mother, the force that wants to keep the child small and dependent. The witch also represents the feeling of wanting to give in to one's laziness, the child's feeling of wanting to eat so many sweets and cake that the witch will later be able to devour him. The child has to learn to form his own opinion and outsmart the witch so that he can develop himself further (*Hansel and Gretel*). This fairy tale contains both female (Gretel) and male (Hans) traits.

The witch also represents the wise old woman who has a special knowledge of nature, herbs and potions, all of which can also be poisonous and can change a person into stone (without growth or feelings).

On the other hand, the good wise woman can help to break the spell. In short, the witch is a special figure, and we have to see when the witch may come to the child or when the child needs to meet the witch. We can help the child by reading fairy tales, but only those in which the wicked witch meets her end by being thrown into a burning cauldron or rolled down the hill in a cask full of nails. Some fairy tales give the wicked old witch a second chance (in a serious talk or a vague promise), but it is actually necessary to be done with that old woman (= old emotion). Otherwise, a child will never be able to make a choice between good and bad, between staying or leaving; he or she will remain on the edge, and the outcome will never be decisive.

A child who is fascinated by the witch may have a conflict with his or her personal mother. However, this conflict may also indicate a necessary phase of growth and taking distance. The wise old woman (who lives in the woods and who knows the secrets of nature) also means that the child has contact with nature and with the magic and magical thoughts that are in keeping with the ages between five and ten. If an older child, far beyond the magical phase, remains fascinated by the witch, this may be an indication of an unresolved conflict from the magical phase. Drawing or playing with the witch is a means of confronting the child again and again with this figure, and we can help the child by trying to see if the witch is helping the child move to a following phase or if the child needs to use his strong points to free himself of the witch.

4. Magicians

A child who is difficult to reach and who rejects those who try to come into contact with him is often a child who shows few emotions. The magician is the suitable figure here because the magician is the invisible figure who lives as a hermit in a castle or on a mountain top but who nevertheless has power over the people who try to visit him since the bad magician is able to cast spells and change people into stones. Opposed to this is the good magician, such as Merlin, who possesses wisdom but who will share his wisdom only with those who travel with him. The archetypal and symbolic significance of the magician points to both characteristics.

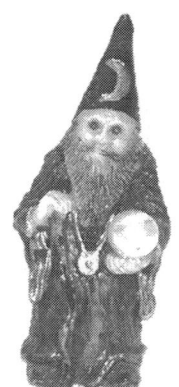

A child who is a bit lonely, aloof or without emotions can be helped by playing with the magician (or as the magician) because it possesses the same traits. As parents, we can help the child by trying to understand both the positive and negative traits of the fantasy figure with whom the child has established a (temporary) friendship. We can also help the child by reading him or her fairy tales in which a magician plays a role (such as King Arthur or Harry Potter).

The magician can be a special friend of the child who is a loner. Because the child is withdrawn into himself, he has an almost invisible power over others because he makes the others powerless. We can try to help this child by listening to the child's 'wisdom'.

5. Dwarves

These little dwarves are special fantasy figures that appeal to children. Dwarves are tiny men who live in the woods where they work in underground mines searching for diamonds. Dwarves perform tasks for people in need if they cannot do the work themselves. They are creative and inventive. Children (and intuitive adults) are able to listen to dwarves since dwarves represent intuitive little voices that tell you what you should or should not do. The bond with nature is the dwarves' most characteristic trait. But there are also disgusting dwarves who are always in a bad mood (for example, Grumpy in *Snow White and the Seven Dwarves*). According to M.L. van Franz, the irritability of some dwarves is the shadow side of creativity. If creativity cannot be expressed, a person becomes bad-tempered and irritable (*Zeitschrift für Sandspieltherapie* Vol.13, p. 17). We can also encounter these irritable dwarves in artists when they find themselves in a phase of uncertainty in their creative process. The very question 'What is this going to be?' will cause them to walk off in anger!

This phase of uncertainty can also be experienced by a child who is approaching a process of change in his development. In a therapeutic process, we can see this happening when there are indications that the child is ready for changes in behaviour and emotions. This is often accompanied by a phase of irritability, which some therapists refer to as 'resistance'.

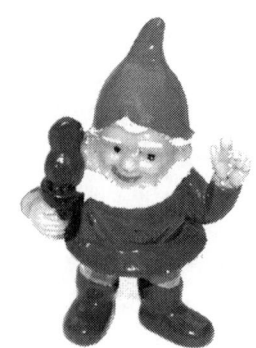

It is worth noting that dwarves are again getting a great deal of attention in today's world. In almost all Western countries that are characterized by technology and over-population, dwarves can be found in all sorts of gardens, ranging from terraced houses in an English suburb to the large villas in Switzerland, the United States and Canada. This phenomenon may be an indication of the universal human need to remain in touch with the natural and creative aspects of being human.

Children and dwarves belong together. Children and dwarves play, dance and have fun. We show children the wonders of nature and teach them the names of flowers, trees and animals. We take children in search of dwarves who secretly do our work for us. The dwarves are present if we teach the child to listen to his 'own nature' by letting him do things in his own way, with improvisation and pleasure. This means that we have to give the child freedom, that we should not make rules about creativity but should let the child discover his own creativity.

The angry dwarf does need some support and may perhaps need to be helped (but the angry dwarf in fairy tales is never thankful). In most cases, it is usually better to give him a wide berth, to let him 'stew in his own juices'.

6. Clowns

We finally come to the figure of the clown, the figure who wears of mask of ambivalence because he laughs and cries at the same time. He makes fun of the world and acts as if he is stupid. Meanwhile, however, he is showing people a reflection of themselves. The clown falls into the category of jokers, jesters, harlequins and buffoons.

The clown is the archetype of the person who feels himself to be different, a feeling of loneliness that arises because he has no normal relationship with those around him. The clown points to a feeling of being unloved. He amuses others but keeps his own emotions hidden. A child who plays the clown may feel lonely or excluded or may have difficulty making normal contact with 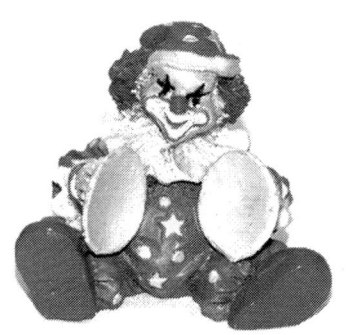 those around him. These children are often well aware of another's weak points, they can imitate others easily and make fun of them, but they show little of their own emotions. Such a child can be helped by having him express his own emotions. He or she must learn to deal with sadness and pleasure, power and powerlessness. These feelings should be experienced and not transformed into a game of playing the clown in which the child puts on a mask.

The clown also shows us that we should not take life too seriously and that we should learn to enjoy laughing and to see humour in small things. The clown also teaches us that we should put mistakes, human aberrations and ostentation into perspective.

It is quite usual in today's hospitals to entertain seriously ill children with visits from the 'clinic-clowns' The circus clown with his white face, his big red mouth and his black eyes is a ghostly figure connected with death, but also a figure who, with his feet in their oversized shoes firmly planted on the ground, is not afraid of anything. At the children's ward of a hospital, the clown ensures that serious things such as operations and painful treatments can be joked about so that the child's fear of such things diminishes.

(The fantasy figures in the photographs in this chapter are between 5 cm and 8 cm tall and form part of my collection of miniatures for Sandplay therapy. T.F.)

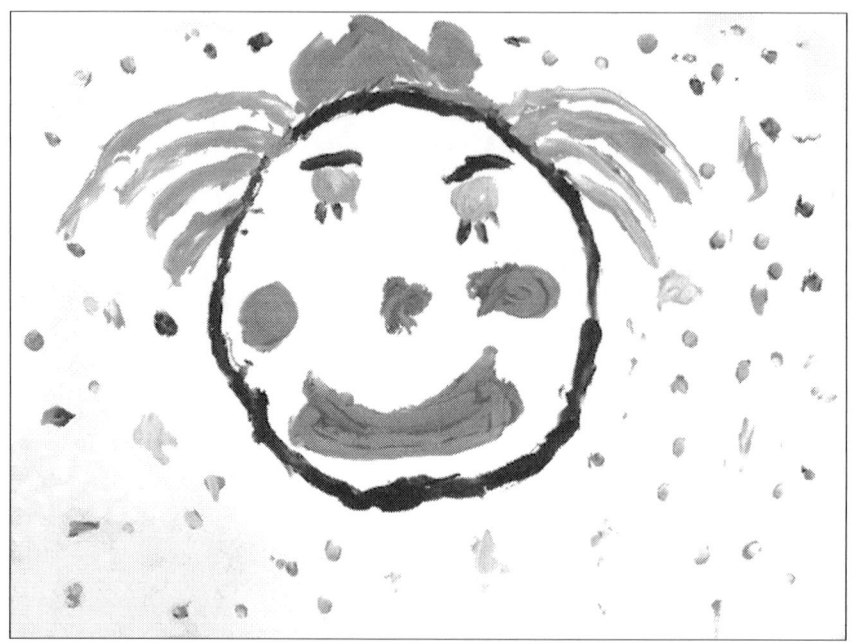

the clown (boy, eight years old)

In this way, children give signals in their drawings and in their games. They ask questions and give answers to the questions that they themselves pose.

Fantasy figures that are in fashion or are popular with children because there are TV series, computer games or books about them refer to archetypal feelings. This is true of knights, queens, Indians, Pocahontas and Alladin and of the more contemporary Pokemon, Power Rangers, Harry Potter and all those who play a role in these popular stories.

We can share the child's feelings if we are able to appreciate the deeper significance of this symbolic language. Animals and fantasy figures are archetypes that offer help in effecting the necessary growth of the self-conscious. And these archetypes are found not only in drawings but also in all sorts of games, in stories, music, dance and daily life. We can learn these again from children if we spontaneously dare to play as a child.

CHAPTER 11

INTERPRETING DRAWINGS

11.1 Learning to look at children's drawings

In order to understand the significance of children's drawings, we have devoted the previous chapters to a detailed study of the general and universal development of drawings made by children. We have tried to show what a drawing signifies in a certain phase for a certain child. It was not the intention, nor is it possible, to suggest that a drawing can be a complete diagnostic aid once we know its significance. Personal experiences, cultural and family circumstances and physical factors also play a role, all of which are expressed in the drawing. Some of these factors are known, others are unknown and still others are in the realm of the subconscious. We are unable to fully fathom the subconscious of either the creator of the drawing or the viewer.

A drawing is not a test, but it is a *means of communication*. The previous chapters were intended to give the reader insight into the development of children's drawings (and children's games) and the relationship between this development and the growth of the psyche. Following our children's development is a rich experience that brings us into contact with the source of man's creative powers. As children, we once followed the path of our ancestors and we recognize this again in children's drawings. The development of a child is a reflection of man's prehistory, the child's own personal development and all that the child, as a member of the next generation, will contribute to the history of mankind. The child *says something* in his or her drawing, and we can use the universal and symbolic significance of this language of expression to 'understand' what the child is saying. This language has no words, but we can put words to it.

11.2 Drawings and signals

To understand a child's drawing and to recognize any possible special signals, it is very important to be familiar with the *normal* development of drawings at every phase of a child's life. We have studied the *universal* development of children's drawings. In the preceding chapters, we have discussed the significance of the first drawings containing boundlessness, the oval, the spiral and the circle. We then saw that the child began to depict his or her world by drawing people, animals, trees and houses. Colours, forms and stories appeared on the paper as fantasy and reality alternated with each other.

The significance of the drawings was studied in the context of the child's age and accompanying psychological development. As parents, teachers, care providers and therapists, we can better understand children if we are able to recognize the universal, normal and healthy growth of the psyche as is reflected in children's drawings. Only then can we later discern personal signs that may be signals of something unusual, signs and signals that deviate from or do not fit in with a certain phase of life. The language of images is a visual language; to gain insight, we must look. We know this language of images because we too used it as children although we never put this language into words. And words fail here because there is always an aspect of symbolic significance that remains unconscious and can thus never be expressed in words.

We are sometimes aware that a certain drawing says something about a child and his or her personal circumstances. When looking at a child's drawing, we may see signs that call for our attention, signs that have been discussed at length in the preceding chapters. Of course, when looking at a child's drawing, our personal feelings are important, but they reflect our own experiences and feelings and may not be the same as those of the child.

It is not necessary and certainly not correct to try to find a hidden message in a drawing. It is important that we do not give the child the impression that we know more than he or she does about the meaning of a drawing. We can, however, show both understanding and our willingness to understand. The child can sense this and will not need to express himself in words or explanations. As the Jungian analyst Jean Shinoda Bolen once said, we can look at a drawing with a 'green thumb' and try to see all that it contains, or we can look with a 'black thumb' and see only negative things.

11.3   Learning to look systematically

We can use various methodologies to study a drawing systematically. Especially those who are not used to looking at an image or a drawing in this way can benefit from practising the use of a systematic analysis. Although we might be able to say a great deal about a drawing, we should refrain from making any definitive comments since, when making a final evaluation, we should also ask questions about other possibilities, questions to which only the child himself knows the (sometimes as yet unconscious) answers. We must not confront the child with our ideas because the answer may not yet be searched for or put into words since it still lies in the future. That is to say that a drawing is part of a process of development. We do not really help the child by teaching him to draw a circle; the child has to discover this himself! We can, however, create circumstances in which the child can make this discovery: for example, by playing in a circle or with a ball or by dancing together.

An analysis of the images can never result in a final evaluation, but it can lead us to investigate whether or not there are problems so that we can try to provide help for the child. We can, for example, give the child certain toys that fit the stage of psychological growth at which the child finds himself (such as creative material to create order, to mess about with, to fight with, etc.)

Of course, we do have a first impression of a drawing, the feeling we have when we look at a drawing. This first impression stems from our feelings and intuition, feelings that stem from the pre-verbal, unconscious and subjective aspects of ourselves. The importance of these functions has already been discussed in this book as have been the dangers of failing to remember that they are projections of ourselves and not of the child who made the drawing.

Once we have determined the subject of a drawing, we can examine the details and try to find a possible connection between them. We must be familiar with the child's actual situation and the situation in his or her family. We must also take the child's phase of developmental psychology into consideration. We look not only at the surface of a drawing but also at the symbolic significance of figures, colours, forms, etc. As we have seen, a deeper significance becomes clear if we recognize these symbols and examine their significance. As stated earlier, there are no mathematical formulas or dictionaries to explain the significance of these symbols, but knowledge of these symbols will help us to reach a deeper understanding of their significance. If a child makes a spontaneous drawing, he does so from his subconscious. Interpretations can help us to recognize symbols, which is especially important for therapists and care providers but also for parents who, of course, know their own child best.

Various systems from a number of therapeutic schools can help us to examine a drawing in detail. Together, they can help us to analyze a drawing and they can give us a framework in which this systematic analysis can take place. These various schools are:

1. Analytical psychology, especially Jung's typology;
2. Art history and Panofsky's theory of four phases (iconology);
3. Creative therapy and Kliphuis's appeal analysis;
4. An investigation of symbolic significance.

1. Jung's typology
The theory of typology was described by C.G. Jung in his book *Psychological Types*. According to this theory, man possesses four different psychological functions:
1. thinking;
2. observing;
3. feeling; and
4. intuiting.

Thinking and observing see things as they are and nothing more. Feeling and intuiting also see these same things but, in addition, they make more use of aspects and possibilities that may be present in something but that have not yet been consciously observed. Usually, one of these four functions is strongly developed in an individual, and that is then the main function which characterizes that individual's view of the world; the other three functions are supporting functions. These four typological functions can be further categorized into extrovert (oriented towards the external world) and introvert (oriented towards the inner world). It is beyond the scope of this book to discuss these theories in depth, but the basic principles can be used in our study of children's drawings. When looking at these drawings, we can use the four above-mentioned functions by translating them as follows:

Thinking: knowing in which phase of development the child finds himself;
Observing: looking at the details of a drawing;
Feeling: experiencing our own emotion (pleasant or unpleasant);
Intuiting: unconsciously observing and thinking.

The first two functions are a question of fact, but the last two functions are more subjective. If a drawing produces a feeling of sadness without this sadness being caused by certain facts or by the content of the drawing, the person who is confronted by the drawing should take into account his or her own impression. But subjective interpretations must be voiced with caution since we may be projecting our own feelings onto the child. Only when the person viewing the drawing recognizes and admits his or her own feelings rather than projecting them onto the child can the observer's own intuition play a role in empathizing with the child.

2. The theory of phases and iconology

Another way of objectively looking at a drawing is derived from iconology, that branch of science that is devoted to studying the deeper meaning and content of art. The art historian Erwin Panofsky developed a theory to analyze a work of art which consisted of the following four phases:

1. pure summing up of everything that we see (without making any connections between all of these details);
2. naming the subject (connecting the details we have observed with one another);
3. the deeper significance or content of the work of art;
4. asking why the object was made as it was and what the artist intended.

This approach to analyzing an image or a drawing is especially suitable for studying children's drawings that contain a certain subject or that tell a story. It is often useful to practice this approach by, for example, looking at a well-known art object and answering the question phase by phase. Good examples of such analyses can be found in the literature on iconology. In Panofsky's book *Iconological Studies*, he gives the example of Roelof van Straten's iconological analysis of Vermeer's painting *Woman*

Holding a Balance. One of his admonitions is that we should try to think logically and creatively at the same time (p.68)

3. The appeal analysis

The appeal analysis is based on the Freudian theory of phases that was developed in the 1970s by M. Kliphuis, who taught in the programme for creative therapists at Middeloo, (nowadays the University of Professional Education in Amersfoort/Utrecht, The Netherlands.) The underlying theoretical assumptions for this form of analysis can be found in *Het Creatief Proces* (H. Smitskamp and J. ter Velde, 1988). The original appeal analysis is an analysis of the contents of the expression in creative material. The content of an image is analyzed on the basis of thirty-two points that could belong to a certain phase in a child's development. These thirty-two points can be subdivided into six phases of development that are similar to the (Freudian) phases of development from childhood to adulthood.

The phases are as follows:

1. Phase of: feeling boundless, all-powerful, oriented towards one's self, encompassing and armoured (prenatal phase);
2. Phase of: patting, feeling, loneliness, passiveness and receptiveness (passive-oral phase);
3. Phase of: biting, grabbing, tearing, deforming and repairing (active-oral phase);
4. Phase of: smearing, cleaning, conforming, rebelling, conquering opposition, pelting, possessing and retaining (anal phase);
5. Phase of: cleaving, exhibiting, rivalling, making powerless, taking the initiative and becoming independent (latent phase, adolescence);
6. Phase of: producing, repeating and giving (adulthood).

In an appeal analysis, the above are given a value on a seven-point scale, depending on how much a certain aspect is present in or absent from the image. Those appeal elements that are absent represent the forms that have been repulsed. In a therapeutic process, the child (the client) is given the opportunity to discover these forms himself as the basic condition for the creative process (Smitskamp, p. 39). Using this appeal analysis to analyze a child's drawing, we can try to determine if the drawing contains certain noticeable characteristics, forms or subjects that are in keeping with a certain phase. We can then see the similarities in the description of the significance of drawings as we have discussed in the previous chapters ranging from the earliest drawings in the prenatal phase to the drawings in the latent phase and adolescence.

4. Investigating the symbolic significance

We can use all four of the above methods to learn how to look at a child's drawing in order to arrive at a deeper interpretation. Jungian analytical psychology gives an extra dimension to the significance of a drawing because it emphasizes symbolic significance. It is possible to investigate the meaning of symbols. In the previous chapters, we discussed the evolutionary inheritance of the psyche that is stored in every child. This inheritance is also referred to as the 'collective unconscious'. Feelings that rise from the subconscious are symbolically expressed in non-verbal forms of expression such as drawing and other forms of what has been referred to here as 'healing art'.

The development of the child's psyche is expressed in universal symbols in the drawings made by children from early childhood to adolescence. The significance of these symbols has been discussed per age group in the previous chapters.

If a parent, teacher or care provider sees a special detail in a drawing and wants to find its symbolic significance, he or she can do research on symbols as explained in the first chapter of this book. Such a search will always result in special facts, such as a certain knowledge of nature and human history, myths and stories from other cultures and religions, and old and modern fairy tales. The symbols then come to life and bring us into contact with the deeper layers of our own psyche. It can even be the beginning of a new personal process of becoming conscious.

Becoming conscious of one's self is a process that every individual goes through in the course of a lifetime and one which leads to individuation that can be described as 'becoming who you are' or 'realizing all that is in you as fully as possible'. In other words, individuation is a process of growth that leads to adulthood, just as a chestnut becomes a chestnut tree, a calf becomes a cow and a foetus becomes an adult human being. In terms of the growth of the psyche, individuation means a process of differentiation, a process in which an individual becomes aware of his uniqueness. He discovers that which makes him different from his contemporaries. He discovers himself. A person who is himself can live for himself and give others that which they need.

11.4 Let me draw you a picture

The subject of this study, the significance of children's drawings, ends with adolescence. This is not because drawing or other forms of artistic expression stop or that playing games no longer has any significance after childhood. On the contrary, many adults enjoy returning to and refreshing themselves in the paradise of childhood so that they can continue their lives with renewed vigour. Children's drawings are interesting because they not only reflect the development of children but they also bring us – as adults – into contact with the child within ourselves with all its creativity and spontaneity. In a period of difficulty, we can come into contact with this child by playing, drawing, dancing or singing because this 'healing art' has long helped man to express and master his fears. Many adults use 'healing art' to express those very feelings that cannot be put into words. If we are speechless from sorrow from joy, words do not suffice. We then have to dance, jump, write poetry, sing, paint, sculpt and especially … draw!

Nuenen, December 2006

References

Axline, Victoria (1982) *Dibs in Search of the Self.* Penquin Books, London.
Amatruda, Kate (1997) *Sandplay, The Sacred Healing: A Guide to Symbolic Process.* Trance, Sand-Dance Press (USA).
Amman, Ruth (1987*) Traumbild Haus.*Walter-Verlag, Olten.
Amman, Ruth (1989) *Heilige Bilder der Seele. Das Sandspiel, der Schöpferische Weg der Persönlichkeitsentwicklung.* Kösel Verlag, München. (Translated in English (1991) *Healing and Transformation in Sandplay.* LaSalle, Illonois: Open Court.
Bach, Susan (1990) *Life paints his own span.* Daimon Verlag, Zwitserland.
Banning, Cees (1999) *De kinderen van Stenkove.* NRC Handelsblad 24 april 1996.
Baumgardt, Ursula (1990) *Kinderzeichnungen. Bilder der Seele* Kreuz Verlag Stuttgard
Bly, Robert (1992) *Iron John. A Book about Men.* Vintage Books, USA.
Bolen, Jean Shinoda (1984) *Goddesses in Every woman: A new psychology of Women* HarperCollins Publishers USA,
Bowlby, John (1951) *Child care and the growth of love.* London: Penguin
Bowlby, John (1979) *The making and braking of affectional bonds.* Tavistock,
Bradway, Kate (1997*) Silent Workshop of the Psyche.* Routledge (USA).
Bühler, Charlotte (Prof. Dr.) (1937) *Praktische Kinderpsychologie.* Lorenz, Wien.
Cox, Maureen, V. (1993) *Children's Drawings of the human figure* Hove, Erlbaum
Campbell, Joseph (1994) *The Hero With a Thousand Faces.* Bollingen Foundation Inc., N.Y.
Campbell, Joseph en Moyers, Bill (1991) *The Power of Myth* Anchor Books USA
Campbell, Don G. (1997) *The Mozart Effect.* Avon Books, New York.
De Leo, Joseph H. (M.D.) (1973*) Children's Drawings as Diagnostic Aids.* Brunnel/Mazel, USA
Estés, Clarissa Pincola (2003) *Women who Run with the Wolves* Ballantine Books
Einstein, Albert (1954) *Ideas and Opinions. Based on Mein Weltbild, edited by Carl*
Seelig and orther sources. New translations and revisions by Sonja Bargmann. Wings Books, New York, (Part V, 290 e.v.)
Escher, M.C. (1992) *Escher: Life and Work* H.N.Abrams. London
Erikson, Erik H. (1962) *Childhood and Society* Norton Company Inc. New York
Eschenbach, U (Hrsg) (1978) *Das Symbol im therapeutische Prozesz bei Kinder und Jugenlichen.* Verlag Adolf Bonz, GmbH, Stuttgart.
Ferenszi, Sandor (1988) *Het oceanische gevoel* Boom, Meppel/Amsterdam. (original text: *Versuch einer Genitaltheorie.(*(1924) Psychoanalytischer Verlag Leipzig/Wien
Fleck-Bangert, Rose (1995) *Kinderen setzen Zeichen* Köser Verlag& Co. München.
Fontana, D. (1993) *The secret language of symbols. A visual key to symbols and their meanings.* Paviljon, London.
Fowler, John en Ardon A.M. *The Diagnostic Drawing series and Dissociative disorders; a Dutch study,* 2001. (Cohen, B.M. (Ed.) The Diagnostic
Drawing Series, Revised Rating Guide.
Franz, Marie-Louise (1974) *Problems of the feminine in fairytales.* Spring Publ. New York
Franz, Marie-Louise (1974) *Shadow and Evil in fairytales* Spring, Zürich.
Franz, Marie-Louise (1990) *Individuation in Fairy Tales.* Shambhala Publications, London.
Franz, Marie-Louise (1996) *Interpretation of Fairy Tales* Shambala Prod. Boston
Franz, Marie-Louise (1998) *C.G. Jung. His Myth in OurTime.* Inner City Books, Canada.
Franz, Marie-Louise (1978) In: *man and his Symbols.* Pan Books Ltd. London (p.230)
Freud, Sigmund Prof. Dr. (1991) *Introductory Lectures on Psychoanalysis* Penguin Books London
Freud, Anna (1991) *The Ego and the mechanisms of Defense* Karnac Books, New Ed. edition
Fraiberg, Selma H. (1996) T*he Magic Years. Understanding and handling broblems of early chilhood.* Fireside New York

Friedman, Harriet (1997) *Eine Sicht des Sandspiels*. Zeitschrift für Sandspiel Therapie (Heft 7 Verlag Linde v. Keyserlingk, Stuttgart (transl. lecture August 22 1996. into German (*Bridging Analytical Psychology and Research: A Sandplay View*) at the International Congress for Analytical Psychology IAAP, Los Angelos).
Fromm, Erich (1960) *Fear for freedom*. Routledge & Kegan Paul. New York
Furth, Gregg, M. (1988)) *The Secret World of Drawings*. Sigo Press, Boston
Gay, Peter (1988) *Freud: A Life for our times*. Norton, New York
Glyn, Thomas V en Silk, Angele M.J. (1990) *An introduction to the psychology of children's drawings*. Harvester Wheatsheaf, New York.
Graetz, H.R. (1963) *The Symbolic Language of Vincent van Gogh*. New York-Toronto-Londen.
Grimm, Jacob en Willem (1909) *The fairy tales of the Brothers Grimm*. Constable, London.
Grof, S. Bennett H.Zina (1992) *The holotropic Mind: three levels of human consciousness and how they shape our lives* HarperSanFrancisco. San Francisco.
Hall James (1994) *Hall's Illustrated Dictionary of Symbols in Eastern and Western Art*. John Murray (Publishers) London.
Heller, E. (1990) *Kleur, symboliek, psychologie en toepassing*. Het Spectrum, Utrecht.
Hellendoorn, Joop (red.) (1988) *Therapie, kind en spel*. Van Loghum Slaterus, Deventer.
Hellendoorn, Joop (1992) *Beeldcommunicatie, een vorm van kinderpsychotherapie*. Bohn Stafleu van Loghum, Deventer.
Herder Lexicon (1986) *The Herder symbol dictionary*, ed. by B. Matthews, Wilmette III, Chiron.
Horney Karen (1993) *Feminine psychology*. W.W. Norton Company, New York-London.
Itten, Johannes (1970) *The elements of color* Whiley and Sons.
Jung, Carl, G. (1968)) *The Archetypes and the Collective Unconscious (1986) Reprinted, second edition, C.W., part 1*. Routlegde London.
Jung, Carl, G. (1978) *Man and his Symbols*. Pan Books Ltd. London
Jung, Carl, G. (1987) *Beelden uit mijn leven*. Lemniscaat, Rotterdam.
Jung, Carl, G. (1991) *Kinderdromen*. Lemniscaat, Rotterdam.
Jung, Carl, G. (1995) *Psychologie und Alchemie*. Walter-Verlag, Solothurn-Düsseldorf.
Jung, Carl, G. (2003) *Psychologische typen*. Lemniscaat, Rotterdam.
Kalff, Dora (1966) *Sandspiel: Seine therapeutische Wirkung auf die Psyche*. Rentsch, Zurich.
Kalff, Dora (1980) *Sandplay, a psychotherapeutic approch to the psyche*. Sigo Press, Boston.
Kast, Verena (1995) *Folktales as therapy* Fromm Int.
Kellogg, Rhoda (1969) *Analyzing Children's Art*. Mayfield Publishing Company.
Kielig, W.(1978) *Volken en stammen*(Red. Jo Brücke ep Büttinghausen) Amsterdam Boek.
Kiepenheuer, Kasper (1990) *Crossing the Bridge: A Jungian Approach to Adolescence*. Open course Publishing, New York.
Kiepenheuer, Kasper (1989) *Was Kranke Kinder Sagen Wollen*. Kreuz Verlag
Klein, Melanie (1983) *Die Psychoanalyse des Kindes*. (reprint Klett-Cotta) Stuttgart.
Kliphuis, Maks (Wils, Rex red.) (1979) *Bij wijze van spelen. Creatieve processen bij vorming en hulpverlening*. Samson Uitgeverij Alphen a.d. Rijn/Brussel.
Koch, Karl (1982) *Der Baumtest Der Baumzeichenversuch als psychdiagnostisch Hilfsmittel*. Verlag Hans Huber (9. korr. Auflage).
Kris, E. (1952) *Psychoanalytic explorations in Art*. International University Press, New York
Kübler-Ross, Elisabeth (1981) *Living with Death and Dying*. MacMillan, New York.
Kübler-Ross, Elisabeth (1983) *On Children and Death*. MacMillan, New York.
Leo Di, Joseph H, M.D.(1973) *Children's Drawings as Diagnostic Aids* Brunner/Mazel, New York
Lewis, Penny en Bernstein, Penny (1994) *Theoretical Approaches in Dance-Movement Therapy*. Routledge, USA.
Lüscher, M. (1971) *Der Lüscher Test, Persönlichkeitbeurteilung durch Farbwahl*. Reinbek.
Lucker. Manfred (1991) *Wörterbuch der Symboliek*. Alfred Kröner Verlag Stuttgart.
Malchiodi, Cathy A. (1998) *Understanding Children's Drawings*. The Guilford Press, New York

Malchiodi, Cathy A. (1997) *Breaking the Silence* (sec.ed.) Brunner-Routledge, New York
Mahler, Margareth S. (2000) *The Birth of the Human Infant: Symbiosis and Individuation.* Basic Books.
Mahler, Margareth S. (2000) Fred Pine, and Annie Bergman *The psychological Birth of the Human Infant.* Basic Books.
Markell, Mary Jane (2002) *Sand, Water, Silence. The embodiment of the Psyche.* Jessica Kingsley Publishers.
Medhananda en Yvonne Artaud (1991) *Der Weg des Horus. Bilder des inneren Weges im alten Agypten.* Bonz Verlag, Fellbach.
Miller, Alice (1981) *The Drama of the Gifted Child. The Search for the True Self.* Basic Book
Miller, Alice (1990) *The Untouched Key. Tracing Childhood Trauma in Creativity and Destructiveness.1 Doubleday. 1st. Anchor Books.*
Miller, Alice (1990) *Hidden Cruelty in Child-Rearing and the Roots of Violence.* Farrar Straus & Giroux..
Mitchell, R en Friedman, H. (1994*) Sandplay*: *Past, Present en Future.* Routledge London.
Morris Desmond (1962) *The biology of Art.* New York: A.A. Knopf
Navone Andreina (1998) The *Double Birth: The Clinical Story of Emanuele.* Journal of Sandplay Therapy. Volume VII, Number I, 1998.
Neumann, Erich (1959) *The Archetypal World of Henry Moore.* Harper Torchbook (Bollinger Library).
Neumann, Erich (1973) *The Child, Structure and Dynamics of the Nascent Personality.* Hodder and Stoughton, London, Sydney, Auckland, Toronto.
Neumann, Erich (1974) *Art and the Creativ Unconscious.* Princeton University Press.
Neumann, Erich (1991) *The Great Mother.* Princeton University Press.
Neumann, Erich (1993) *The Origins and History of Consciousness.* Princeton University Press.
Nilsson, Lennart (1986) *A Child is Born.* Dell, revised edition.
Oda, Takao (1997) *Agression and Containment in Sandplay.* Journal of Sandplay Therapy Volume VI, number 2). ISSN 1089-6457 (Walnut Creek, California).
Onian, Richard B. (1951) *The Origins of European Thought about the Body, the Mind, the Soul, the World, Time and Fate.* Arno Press.
Piaget, Jean (2000) *The psychology of the Child.* Basic Books . Reissued .
Panofsky, Erwin (1972) *Studies in iconology; humanistic themes in the art of the Renaissance.* HarperCollins Publishers. New ed.
Pennington, Yvonne Ph.D. USA, dissertatie: *The Sandtray Assessment of Development (SAD).* Presentatie Zwitserland, Ittingen ISST 2001 (*artikel in: wwpsychology.am/index. html).*
Pinker, Peter (1999) *How the mind works.* W.W. Norton & Company.
Riedel, Ingrid (1994*) Hildegard von Bingen, Prohphetin der Kosmischen Weisheit.* Kreuz Verlag, Stuttgart.
Riedel, Ingrid (1992) *Mahltherapie.* Kreuz Verlag, Stuttgart.
Riedel, Ingrid (1983) *Farben in Religion, Gesellschaft, Kunst und Psychotherapie.* Kreuz Verlag, Stuttgart.

Riedel, Ingrid (1985) *Formen, Kreis, Kreuz, Dreieck, Quadrat. Spirale.* Kreuz Verlag, Stuttgart.
Riedel, Ingrid (1991*) Bilder, in Therapie, Kunst und Religion, Wege zur Interpretation.* Kreuz Verlag, Stuttgart.
Rowling, J.K. (1998) *Harry Potter & de Steen der Wijzen.* Uitgeverij De Harmonie, Amsterdam.
Rossiter, Evelyn (1979) *Het Egyptische dodenboek. Beroemde Egyptische Papyri.* Atrium, ICOB Alphen a.d. Rijn.
Royer le, Jacqueline*: Dessin d'une maison, image de l'ádaptation sociale de l'enfant.* (Teken-Een-Mens-test).
Rutten-Saris M. Ph.D. *A Diagnostic instrument for the assessment of interaction structures in*

drawings. *(artikel in :www.eblcentre.com/dutch.right.html)*
Sanders-Woudstra (red.) (1996) *Kinder- en Jeugdpsychiatrie Psychopathologie en behandeling.* Van Gorkum & Comp., Assen.
Schenda, Robert (1998) *Who's is who der Tiere. Märchen, Mythen und Geschichten. Das ABC der Tiere.* Deutsche Taschenbuch Verlag.
Schmeer, G. (1978) *Heilende Bäume. Baumbilder in der psychotherapeutischen Praxis.* Pfeiffer.
Schottenloher, Gertraud (1989) *Wenn Worte fehlen, sprechen Bilder.* Kösel Verlag, München.
Schrauwers G.M. (e.a.) *Pedagogische Platenatlas.* Pax.Uitg. Den Haag.
Schretlen, Ignace (2003) *Over de wortels van creativiteit. Onderzoek naar krabbels van mensapen en peuters. Kunstje of oorsprong van kunst?* (artikel in: www .iaaa.nl-/cursusAA&A1/Schretlen).
Sigg, Eva (2001) *Penelope und Odysseus (Ein getrenntes Paar auf dem Wege zur Wiedervereinigung und zur inneren Ganzeit.)* Eigen Uitgave, Willikon/Zürich
Schoeman, Stan (2003 Internet) *Eloquent beads, the semantic of a ZULU art form.* (artikel in: www.minotaur.images.co.za/client/zulu/bead.html)
Smitskamp, H en Tervelde J. (red.) (1988) *Het Kreatief Proces.* Phaedon Uitgeverij, Culemborg.
Spock Dr. Benjamin (1968*) Baby- en Kinderverzorging.* Uitgeverij Contact Amsterdam.
Steinhardt, Leonore (2000*) Foundation and Form in Jungian Sandplay.* Jessica Kingsley Pub. London, New York.
Strauss, Michaele (1990) *Kindertekeningen.* Uitgeverij Christofoor.
Strich, Christian (1993) *Het mooiste sprookjesboek.* (verzameld en vertaald) Uitg. Van Reemst, Houten.
Studienzentrum Sandspieltherapie, abteilung Sandspieltherapieforschung: *SAT-Studie Sandspiel Therapie* Dr. C. Senges, Ph.Dr. A. v. Gontard, Im Linsenbühle, 69221 Heidelberg.
Suzuki, D.T (2000) *Inleiding tot het Zen-Boeddhisme.* Ankh Hermes.
Sykes, B.(2002) *De zeven dochters van Eva.* Uitgeverij De Fontein, Amsterdam
Thomas, Glyn V. en Silk, Angele M.J (1993) *De psychologie van kindertekeningen.* Swets & Zeitlinger.
Timmer, Maarten (2001) *Van Anima tot Zeus. Encyclopedie van begrippen uit de mythologie, religie, alchemie, cultuurgeschiedenis en analytische psychologie.* Lemniscaat, Rotterdam.
Vries, A. de (1984) *Dictionary of Symbols and Imagery.* Elsevier, Amsterdam.
Willemsen, Annemarieke (2003) *Romeins speelgoed. Kindertijd in een wereldrijk.* **Walburg Pers Zutphen.**
Willis, Roy (red.) (2000) *XYZ van de Mythologie. Goden, godinnen, helden, heldinnen en legendarische dieren verklaard.* (Oorspronkelijke titel: Dictionary of World Myth, by Duncan Baird Publishers, London) Uitg. Areopagus.
Wils, Rex (1979) *Bij wijze van spelen, creatieve processen bij vorming en hulpverlening.* (1[e] druk, 4[e] opl.) Samson Uitg. Alphen a.d.Rijn/Brussel.
Winnicot D.W. (1964) *The child, the family and the outside world.* Penquin Psychology.
Winnicot D.W. (1971) *Playing and reality.* Basic Books.

Wit, Jan (Prof. dr.) en Veer, Guus van der (1991) *Psychologie van de Adolescentie.* INTRO, Nijkerk.
Woodman Marion and Bly Robert (1998) *The Maiden King. The reunion of masculine and feminine.* Henry Holt and Company. Inc.New York.
Wright, Robert (1995) *The Moral Animal: Evolutionary Psychology and Everyday Life.*Vintage Books

Internet

page
1   *www.psychceu.com/trauma.html)* Kate Amatruda, Teaching Member Sandplay Therapist (drawing Martin Gocobachi with permission)
5   *www.skynet.be/sven.gheeraert/oezki5.html (2003) 9 photo (*with permission)
19   *www.darkfiber.com/eyeinhand (2002)*
20   *www.culture.f*
22   *www.teako170.com/graffiti2.html* (2002)
23   *www. literatuurgeschiedenis.nl* (2003)
24   *www.micro.magnet.fsn.edu/creatures/technical/packages.html (2003)*
33   *www.vaktherapie.nl (*Federatie van Vaktherapeutische Beroepen) (2006)
35   *www.isst-society.org* (International Society for Sandplay Therapy)(2006)
-     *www.sandplaynederland.org* (Ned. Vereniging van Sandplay Therapeuten) (2006)
-     *www.psychology.am/index.html* (2003)(Mrs. Pennington).
-     *www.kindertherapie.8m.com* (Office Theresa Foks-Appelman) (2004)
120   *www.warchild.nl (2003)* (War child organisation the Netherlands)(2003)
138   *www.theartgallery.com.au/kidsart.html* (World wide childrens drawings).(2003)
-     *www.childrens-drawing.com/eng/museum.htm* (December 2006) The International Environmental Children's Drawing Contest
163   *www.touregypt.net/featurestories/sphinx1.htm (2006)*

INDEX

A
aboriginals, 9, 57, 58
abuse, 16, 49
adolescent, 60, 129, 153
adoption, 16
Aggression, 78, 82, 83, 89, 126
    157-159
alchemists, 4, 8-9, 150
alchemy, 149
Amman Ruth, 35, 96
analytical psychology, 8,12, 28,
    34, 35, 47, 73, 150, 172,
    185
anima /animus, 12, 55
animal, 21, 76-77, 101, 109, 110,
    116, 123, 146, 161 – 169,
    176, 178
  in tree, 161
  symbol of, 7
animalistic phase, 161-167
appeal analysis, 33, 182
archetypal mother, 49, 52, 96,
156-   159
art modern, 141
art therapy, 20, 33, 47
artist. 117, 129, 136, 142, 162,
    175, 183
attachment,49
autistic, 92

B
balloons, 61
Barbie doll, 172
basic forms, 64, 71, 151
belly, 73, 114
bible, 6, 53, 144
Bingen Hildergard, von, 148
biological birth, 27,46

bird
  - *symbol*, 5-7
black, 137, 141
  - sun 100
black, symbol, 146
blue, 133
Bly, Robert, 127
boat, 124-125,140
body painting, 58
Bolen, Shinoda, 108
books of symbols, 7
borderline, 49
Bosch, Hieronymous, 8
bottom, 154 - 156
  edge, 103
boundlessness, 39, 41-
    46, 65, 105, 139,150,
    180, 184
Bowlby, 3, 25, 28
branch , 106-112
breasts, 70,86,158
brown, 110, 149
butterfly, 120
buttons, 83,84

C
Campbell, Joseph, 16
cartoons,.24,117,137,138
case illustration, 88 ,91, 93,
    103,105,110, 111, 112.
    120, 140, 150, 194
cave drawings, 4, 20, 21-23
chaos, 15, 39-40, 57, 149
cheeks, 93
child and mythology 14,
chimney, 96, 99, 104
chip designers 24
circle 43, 46-48, 51-55, 61, 69,
    111, 151, 156, 180 - 181
clay, 4,9, 19, 42, 47, 52, 66, 150

clinic clowns, 177
   see also: clown
clothes, 99, 100-102, 107, 117, 145, 158
clown, 176, 177, 178
collective unconscious, 11, 12, 34, 133, 156, 162, 164, 185
colouring books, 67, 68
colours, 64, 67, 138
   - symbolic, 141 – 150
computer, 5, 22, 137, 139
   -games, 123, 152, 171
   -drawing, 137
    micro chips, 24
constant object, 3, 54
contact disorder, 3
container, 43, 72
corners, 17, 52, 65, 155 – 159
cosmos, 15, 56, 151
Cox, Maureen, 30
creation (of the world) 15, 41
creative arts, 139
Crocodile, 163, 164
Crosses 47, 59, 60,139
Crossroads, 2, 60
crown (of leaves), 198
cube, 152

D

Daedalus., 62
dance, 142
   - therapy, 19,20
decorating (bodies), 58.
depression, 128, 135, 146
details (in clothes), 78
Diagnostic Drawing 30, 33, 179
Dinosaurs, 168,169
Dionysus., 134

direction 39, 59, 94, 152, 155, 156
Disney 67, 170
dog, 106, 169
dots, 50-51, 56 – 58, 74, 83
Draw-A-House, 96, 101, 106
Draw-a-Person, 30, 70
drawing without borders, 38, 51, 151, 152
drawings by boys 122, 123
drawings by girls, 123 e.v.
dreams, 4,5,79, 116, 137, 169
Dutch newspaper, 119
dwarves, 175, 176

E

ears, 81, 88, 91, 97
egg-shaped drawing, 29, 40, 41, 42, 43
Ego, 14, 47, 51,, 79, 84, 91, 167
Ego-consciousness, 53, 58 – 60
egocentricity, 84
Egyption hieroglyphics, 4,60,163
Einstein, Albert, 31
Elves, 171, 172
embryo, 17,18,39,41,43,97
Erikson, Erik H, 25, 28.
Escher, M.C.. 45, 136, 137
Eschenbach, Ursula (Hrsg) ,151, 181
evaluation, 30
evolution, 17, 26, 69, 70, 78,. 82, 122
eyes, 71, 73 – 74, 79, 80, 97, 98, 120
eyes and hands, 19

F

face, 40, 52, 79, 88, 115, 117
fairy, 13, 172, 173
faeces, 66, 75, 140, 149
fairy tales, 7, 16, 20, 60, 79, 123
— 124, 135, 162, 169 – 176, 185
family as an animal, 163
fantasy, 32, 67, 113, 138, 161, 170, 180
fantasy figures, 35, 169- 175, 177, 178
fence, 99, 101, 128, 151
Finger paint drawing, 56, 65, 66
Fingers, 81, 82, 91
  - *nails*, 82
first impression, 88, 91, 181
fish-like, 17, 43
five, 82
Fleck Bangert, Rose, xiv, 54,, 59
foot *(feet)* 77, 82, 83
Fraiburg Selma, 76
Franz, M.L. von, xiv, 7, 48, 156, 175,
Freud, S., 4, 11, 30, 32, 39, 44, 72, 75, 114, 184
Freud, Anna, 25
Fromm, Erich, 14, 26
front door, 99
fruit, 109, 110, 147, 167
Furth, Gregg, 33

G

games, 32, 46, 47, 52, 62, 66, 75, 117, 121, 132, 139, 178
 -*computer*, 123, 152, 170, 171, 178
 -*war*, 127
genitals 75, 86 – 89
Gilgamesh 48
Glyn, Thomas, 30

Goddess, 13, 14, 144, 145, 148
Gods, 5, 10, 14, 15, 22, 56, 86, 145,
gold, 9, 145, 149, 150
graffiti, 22, 23
grave (stones), 5, 45
green, 120, 121, 128, 143, 147, 148
Grimm, Br., 7, 20, 60, 124, 135
Grof, Stanislav, 41
group awareness, 121

H

hair, 38, 79, 85, 88, 91, 92
handicap, 53
hands, 19, 35, 68, 81, 82, 89, 93
Hansel and Gretel, 173
hat, 85, 88
head, 71, 72 – 74, 78, 79, 91, 98. 162, 163
headgear, 85
healing art, 20, 129, 136, 185, 186
hieroglyphics
  see: Egyptian
History
  - *human/evolution*, 7, 8, 14, 18, 32, 69, 72, 107, 122, 130, 164, 179, 185
  - *drawing/art*, 20, 23, 30, 34, 115, 116, 155, 182
  - *consciousness*, 12, 15, 31
hole, 198, 109
horse, 3, 32, 109, 123, 124
house, 95, 98, 102 0 105, 120
  - *walls*, 96- 98, 104, 105
  - *windows*, 29, 98, 97, 103,- 105, 114
  - *front door*, 99
  - *surrounding*, 99

- *roof*, 96, 97, 102 – 105, 120, 153, 198

I
I-awareness, 47, 49, 51
Icarus, 62
iconology, 182, 183
impressionists, 9
individualization, 16, 48
  -*and separation*. 25, 54, 64,
industrial revolution, 18, 32
inner child, 150
instincts, 2, 16, 48, 77, 107, 122, 142, 161, 165 - 169
Internet, 24, 138
interpreting, 12, 31, 159, 179 - 186
intuition, 15, 31, 60, 181, 183
ISST, 35
Itten, Johannes, 143

J
judicial evidence, 102, 107
Jung C.G. 4, 7, 9, 11, 16, 18, 30, 48, 69, 151, 156, 164, 182
Jungian analytical therapy, 12, 26, 34, 47, 55, 149, 150, 157, 185

K
Kalff, Dora, 3, 4, 35, 168, 170
Kast, Verena, 7, *135*
Kellogg, Rhoda, 29, 30, 69, 95
Kiepenheuer, Kasper, 33, 131, 135
King Arthur, 48, 175
Klein, Melanie, 32
Kliphuis M., 33, 182, 184
knees, 83, 93,

Koch, Karl, 106
Kohnstam, 84
Kris, Ernst, 167
Kübler-Ross, Elisabeth, 33

L
labyrinth, 152
Lady Di,, 16
latency phase, 113

M
mother
  - *archetype*, 12, 26,
  - *and child*, 25 – 28, 41, 46, 50, 83, 84, 131, 153
  - *Earth/Nature*, 13, 149, 131, 133
  - *Great the*, 12, 13, 14, 21 156, 159
  - *personal*, 100, 173, 174
    see also: *archetypal mother*
mouth, 19, 52, 72, 78 – 80, 88, 92, 93, 97, 177
mud, 66
music, 32, 46, 120, 129, 133, 136, 139 – 140
  -therapie, 28, 47
mythology, 6, 12, 14, 16, 20, 62, 79, 84, 144 – 145

N
Navrone, Adreina, 28
narrative drawing, 116, 119, 157, 158
navel, 83 – 84, 91 – 92
  -stone, 84
neck, 81, 89, 91, 93,
nest, 63, 109, 122, 161, 163

Neumann, Erich, xiv, 12, 14, 15, 21, 26, 34, 69, 101
Nilsson Lennart, 17
nose, 57, 73, 80
nucleus, 40, 41

O
observing, 31, 182, 183
oceanic feeling, 39
Odysseus, 125 – 126
oedipal, 11, 114
Onians, Richard, 83
oral, 72, 88, 89,. 93, 184
orange, 103, 120, 121, 146, 148, 149
original (drawing), 137

P
Panofsky, 182, 183
paradise, 2, 14, 43, 113, 131, 166
Pegasus, 124
phallus, 86
Pennington, Yvonne, 35
perspective, 102, 115, 116, 126, 136 – 138, 151, 156, 159
philosophical stone, 5
Piaget, 3, 26, 30 54, 114
Pinkers, Steven, 69
Pinkola, Estes Clarissa, 7
plane (air), 5, 6, 61, 63, 116, 119, 158, 159
play therapy, 26, 33
planet, 15,
poetry 17
Potter, Harry, 5, 16, 48, 175, 178
potty-training, 65, 66, 74, 75, 149,
prehistoric

- cave, 20, 21, 23
- man, 21
prenatal phase, 39, 44, 184, 185
  -feelings, 41
  - memories, 42
pre-school, 7, 29, 42, 44, 62, 76, 84, 100, 101, 146
pre-verbal, 18, 19, 169, 181
primitive people, 15, 17, 56, 58, 86, 97, 131- 133, 164
private parts, 89
process of individuation, 8, 27, 185
  see also: *separation*
proportion, 82, 89, 91 – 94, 108, 110, 113
psyche
  - and body, 17, 8=72, 78, 99, 156, 178
psychopaths, 49
puberty, 37, 85, 113, 121, 125, 129, 138 – 140
pupil (eyes) 80,
purple, 105, 148

R
rainbow, 118
red, 144, 148 - 150, 158
religion, 6, 8, 12, 14, 34, 73, 79, 83, 86, 132, 134, 143, 153, 157, 163, 185
Renaissance, 8, 32
Riedel, Ingrid, xiv, 34, 97, 106, 143, 148, 151, 152, 155
right, 19, 55, 59, 80, 88, 94, 110, 154 – 156, 159
rituals, 13 – 20, 35, 47, 129 – 136
roof, 108 – 110, 158
  see also: *house*
Rowling, J., 5

Royer, le Jacqueline, 96, 102
Rutten-Saris index, 33

S

sadness, 78, 118, 146, 148, 159, 177, 183
sandplay therapy, 18, 20, 28, 34, 35, 170
Schmeer, Gisela, 106
scribble, 3, 29, 37, 38, 70, 105, 139
sculptors, 5
sculpture, 4, 89
Self, the, 9, 47 – 49, 53, 99, 156, 178
separation 27, 28, 50, 54, 55, 64
  see also: individuation
sex, 2, 44, 84, 85,
sexuality, 79, 86, 87, 89
sexual differences, 75, 114, 121
sexual identity, 86, 130
shoes, 82, 83, 89, 93, 177
Sigg, Eva, 125
sign, 144
smell, 18, 72, 80
Smitskamp, H, en ter Velde, J., 33, 184
smoke, 99, 104
snake-like, 1, 43, 44
Snow White, 175
Sobek, God, 163
sperm, 17, 61, 62
sphinx, 163, 162
spiral, 45 – 47, 51, 52, 69, 70, 139, 151, 180
spirituality, 34
spontaneous drawing, 19 68, 117, 182
square, 75, 80, 96 – 99, 151, 152, 157
squirrel, 110

stone, 4,5,9, 14, 22, 84, 148, 149, 158, 174
storytelling, 20
stuffed toy, 76, 161, 165 – 167
sun, 54 – 56, 63, 85, 94, 100, 101, 105, 116 – 120, 142, 145, 147, 149, 158
 - glasses, 100, 116, 158
 - rays, 53, 54, 100,129
surroundings
  and drawing, 89, 92, 94, 96, 99 01, 109, 116, 118, 159
Susan Bach, 33, 142, 1
Suzuki, D.T., 34
Sykes, Brian, 164
symbiotic phase, 27, 49, 50
symbol word, 4
    see also: *house, tree, drawings, animals, colours*

T

tadpole, 69 – 73, 78, 80, 139, 161
tattoos, 58
teddy bear, 165, 166
teeth, 78, 100, 158
therapeutic effect, 33 – 35, 106
therapist, 20, 32, 96, 97, 136, 150, 168, 170, 176, 180, 182
 - creative art, xiii, 33, 120, 184
 - sandplay, 38, 167, 168
three
 - number 98, 153
 - dimensional, 80, 155, 170
toddler, 30, 38, 39, 46, 51, 54, 62, 70, 76, 84, 100, 101, 107, 146, 166, 171
toes, 82, 91
Tolan Patrick H, 130

top, 55, 59, 79, 84, 88, 98, 115, 154, 155, 158
totem, 32, 52, 127, 144, 146, 161, 166, 181
traumatic, 25, 39, 40, 73, 105, 113 118,, 167, 173, 198
tree, 95 – 112
    see also: *trunk, fruit, animal, roots*
triangle, 89, 98, 151, 153, 158
trunk, 106- 112, 158
Twin Towers, 119
typology, 182

U

umbrella, 118
unconscious, collective
  description, 45
universal drawings, 37, 106
Valakovsky, Hans, 119

V

vase, 13, 75
vegatation, 121, 148, 101
vegetative stage, 49, 101, 161, 167
vulture, 7

W

war, 15, 25, 82. 119, 120, 126, 127
War Child, 120
war games
  see *games*
waeving, 39, 61
white, 137, 141, 146, 147, 150, 171, 177,

Willemsen A, 32
windows, see: *house*
Winnicot, D.W., 34, 74, 166, 26
witch, 13,133, 173, 174
womb, 27, 39, 41 – 45, 62, 96, 114
Woodman, Marian, 7, 16
wounds (in trunk) 108
Wrights, Robert, 69

X

X-ray drawings, 102, 114

Y

yellow, 141, 143 – 149
ying-yang, 146, 171
youth camp, 132

Z

Zen, 34, 35

Made in the USA